THE MINDFUL WAY TO A
GOOD NIGHT'S SLEEP

THE MINDFUL WAY
— *to a* —
Good
Night's
Sleep

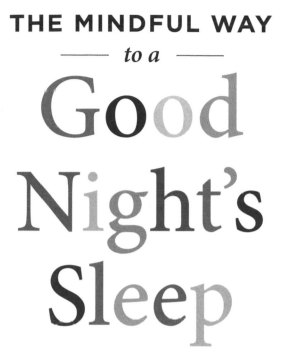

Discover How to Use
DREAMWORK, MEDITATION, and JOURNALING
to Sleep Deeply and Wake Up Well

TZIVIA GOVER

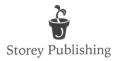

Storey Publishing

The mission of Storey Publishing is to serve our customers by
publishing practical information that encourages
personal independence in harmony with the environment.

EDITED BY Deborah Balmuth, Hannah Fries, and Michal Lumsden
COVER DESIGN BY Alethea Morrison
BOOK DESIGN BY Stacy Wakefield Forte
ART DIRECTION BY Jessica Armstrong
TEXT PRODUCTION BY Jennifer Jepson Smith
INDEXED BY Christine R. Lindemer, Boston Road Communications

COVER ILLUSTRATION BY © ori-artiste/iStockphoto.com
INTERIOR ILLUSTRATIONS BY © Lewis Choong
AUTHOR PHOTOGRAPH BY Carly Rae

Excerpt of "When They Sleep" by Rolf Jacobsen, translation by Robert Hedin,
from *The Roads Have Come to an End Now: Selected and Last Poems of Rolf Jacobsen*
(Copper Canyon Press, 2001). Used by permission of Robert Hedin.

Storey Publishing
210 MASS MoCA Way
North Adams, MA 01247
storey.com

Printed in China by Shenzhen Reliance
Printing Co. Ltd
10 9 8 7 6 5 4 3 2 1

LIBRARY OF CONGRESS CATALOGING-IN-
PUBLICATION DATA

Names: Gover, Tzivia, author.
Title: The mindful way to a good night's sleep:
   discover how to use dreamwork, meditation,
   and journaling to sleep deeply and wake up
   well / by Tzivia Gover.
Description: North Adams, MA : Storey
   Publishing, 2017. | Includes index.
Identifiers: LCCN 2017030618 (print) | LCCN
   2017036038 (ebook) | ISBN 9781612128832
   (ebook) | ISBN 9781612128825 (pbk. : alk.
   paper)
Subjects: LCSH: Sleep disorders—Popular
   works. | Sleep disorders—Treatment—Popular
   works.
Classification: LCC RC547 (ebook) |
   LCC RC547 .G68 2017 (print) | DDC
   616.8/498—dc23
LC record available at https://lccn.loc.
   gov/2017030618

Dedicated
to all dreamers, everywhere.

CONTENTS

Sleep, sleep, beauty bright,
Dreaming in the joys
of night.

WILLIAM BLAKE,
"CRADLE SONG"

BEDTIME STORY
Talking in My Sleep

I've had a complicated relationship with sleep and dreams from the start. I was that kid who feared the dark and made my parents leave the hall light on and my bedroom door cracked open all night. Even then, I'd lie beneath my floral-print comforter, not feeling at all comforted. I envied the children in Mary Poppins whose nanny sat by their beds, watching over them as they slept. I begged my mother to do the same, but after I'd said my prayers and closed my eyes, she'd retreat with a kiss on the forehead.

Some nights I lay awake listening to the restless creaking of our old house as if it too were having a hard time settling down for the night, and when I'd finally doze off, I'd often be haunted by nightmares. Summers at sleepaway camp, I was infamous for waking my bunkmates when I talked in my sleep. A simple night of easy rest, it seemed, was beyond me.

As adults we may overcome our fears of monsters under the bed and things that go bump in the night, but an atavistic sense of anxiety still clings to many of us like a stubborn shadow when the sun goes down. So it's not surprising that many of us have trouble sleeping, or avoid adhering to a reasonable bedtime. And we've got more than just the comic books and sitcom reruns of years gone by to keep us awake these days. In the 24-7 hyperconnected culture that's grown up around us, the world stays bright with artificial lights that outshine the stars, and websites entice us to visit, shop, or share long after the last neighborhood café or store has shuttered its windows and locked its doors.

It should come as no surprise then that millions of Americans have experienced some form of insomnia, and as a nation we spend billions of dollars each year to address our sleep deficit. Nor can we deny the toll that all this sleeplessness takes on us individually and as a culture. We suffer from lost productivity at work, increases in obesity and anxiety, diminished cognitive function — and the list goes on.

In response, sleep centers are proliferating around the country to diagnose disorders from snoring to apnea, and pharmaceutical companies have created an array of medications to lull us into slumber. It has become all too common for people to pop a pill in the evening, and then bolt through their days clutching cups of coffee or other caffeinated drinks to keep them awake. But rather than rely on pills and potions, we'd do better to dig down to the roots of our rocky relationship with sleep and make real changes for lasting results.

More and more people are coming to realize that we must look within to be healthy and happy. Using mindfulness-based techniques, we can build habits of attention and intention that promote healthy rest and sound sleep. In fact, studies now show that meditation and mindfulness, practices that cultivate present-moment awareness, are as effective as medication in helping people to sleep soundly and dream well. We can thus empower ourselves to wake up to lives of increased fulfillment and joy.

I know, because this has been my path. The restless nights of anxiety and scary dreams that started when I was a child never completely left me. But over time I've learned (often directly from my dreams themselves) that when I turn to face my fears of the dark — nightmare monsters, attackers, phantoms, and all — I gain courage and confidence as I face the rest of my day. I now have occasional nightmares, but I've also enjoyed many more dreams of beautiful landscapes blossoming with fantastical flowers, wise teachers, and experiences of love and bliss. Dreams have become my allies, and I invite sleep as the territory I cross in order to reach them. Now I teach others to pay attention to how they sleep and what they dream so they, too, can befriend the night. When we do so, we can greet with pleasure the dawning of each day.

On the other hand, if we separate night and day, our sleeping and waking lives, we miss out on the ways that one informs the other. If we don't sleep, we miss out on dreams, and dreaming helps us with emotional regulation, memory consolidation, learning, and problem solving, not to mention the reservoirs of creativity, wisdom, and guidance we can tap into when we study our dreams. When we fail to make space for sleep and dreams, we rob ourselves of our richest waking experiences.

So, while most books tackle one or the other, this book will explore sleep, dreams, and waking as a continuous process, in which each state of consciousness flows naturally into the next. We'll use meditation, journaling, and dreamwork (simple techniques to help you listen to and understand your dreams) as part of a holistic approach so you, too, can sleep, dream, and wake to a life of increased meaning and joy.

Whether you sleep like a baby most nights or toss and turn till dawn, whether you remember dreams regularly or are mystified when you recall one at all, I hope this book will help you. Together we'll welcome the wisdom of sleep, in whatever guise it takes: be it a dark sky of forgetfulness, a fully lit cinematic dreamscape, or anything in between.

BEDTIME STORY

Your early memories of sleep may shed some light on your present-day attitudes. What was nighttime like for you as a child? What were your favorite bedtime routines or rituals? Did you have a favorite bedtime story, blanket, or stuffed animal that escorted you to the Land of Nod? Write about it for three to five minutes. (Just enjoy the process, don't worry about grammar, spelling, or style.)

Like all explorers,
we are drawn to discover
what's waiting out there
without knowing yet
if we have the courage
to face it.

PEMA CHÖDRÖN

BEDSIDE MANNER
How to Use This Book

• • • • • • • •

SLEEP ODYSSEY

I dream I'm shooting through the galaxy in a rocket ship, peering through a telescope for a better view of the wonders of outer space. But instead of seeing new stars, I see a strange city skyline where rooftops are adorned with fantastical spiraling antennae that seem to be receiving signals from some unknown sender. At first I'm disappointed to have flown so far from home only to see an earthly city, exotic though it is.

On waking, I found within this dream a metaphor for the journey we take each night into sleep. When we climb into bed and close our eyes, we blast off like astronauts (or in this case *oneironauts*: those who explore dreams) into the strange bright darkness, perchance to encounter new worlds. Eyes closed, tucked into our beds, we rocket to inner realms of consciousness where we can survey the uncharted territory of our dreaming mind.

Which brings me to those dream rooftops festooned with antennae. For me, they represent the way our minds reach into the darkness while we sleep, searching for signals that arrive in the form of dream symbols and stories. And whether we remember our dreams or not, when our nighttime consciousness splashes down onto the shores of morning, we have the chance to wake to that sense of fresh perspective so treasured by travelers of all stripes. (And who knows, we may even return with a handful of moon rocks or stardust in our pajama pockets, as well.)

pack for the journey

Okay, so you're just going to bed, not blasting off to a distant planet, but you are about to wander deep into the wilds of the night, so you'll want to have some essential supplies handy.

A JOURNAL FOR THE JOURNEY. Whether you're an astronaut visiting the moon, or a botanist tramping through a meadow, observation and recordkeeping are essential to the process of exploration and discovery. Any blank book or notebook can serve as your *"sleep and dreams"* journal. I recommend one with spiral binding and stiff front and back covers that form a firm, flat surface for writing when the journal is propped on your knees in bed.

NIGHT LIGHT. Put a dimmer switch on your bedside lamp, or keep a penlight by your bed so you'll have just enough light to record dreams in the night without waking yourself (or your bed partner) into full alertness.

SLEEP SUIT. A journey is always a good excuse to update your wardrobe. So, whether you prefer to sleep in baby doll nighties, boxers, matching pajama sets, or baggy T-shirts and sweats, take a moment to consider whether your sleep duds are up to par. If not, now's a great time to discard any worn-out, uncomfortable, or ill-fitting pajamas and buy something that will make you look forward to suiting up for sleep.

bedside reading

This isn't simply a book to read. This is a book to *do*. Keep it on your bed stand, so you can read a few pages before you snuggle in for the night or before starting your day. Each page will offer a tip, fact, or technique to spark your curiosity and creativity in the service of making night your best time of day. Here are some things to keep in mind as you read.

TAKE A REST. This book is chock full of ideas and new things to consider. But don't tire yourself out trying to do all of them all the time. On the contrary: try one idea at a time, incorporate what works, and leave the rest. Then, come back to these pages again and again to see if something new catches your attention.

REFRESH TIRED ROUTINES. Getting a good night's sleep and having meaningful dreams shouldn't be one more thing to add to your to-do list. Most of the techniques here are aimed at folding meaning and purpose into things you are already doing each night and each morning, from brushing your teeth and changing into your pajamas to choosing what to have for breakfast. Subtle shifts in attitudes or awareness are often all it takes to revive tired routines and imbue them with relevance.

DOCTOR'S ORDERS. In this book we take a mindful, not a medical, approach to sleep, dreams, and waking well. However, there are physiological and psychological issues, some quite serious, that can affect sleep. The exercises, tips, and techniques included here are meant to support you in reaping the benefits of the natural cycle that comprises nearly a third of our lives, but it should not be used as a substitute for your doctor's advice.

· · · · · · · · ·

INTO THE GOOD NIGHT

Throughout this book you'll be offered various exercises and writing prompts to help you improve your relationship with sleep and dreams. Following are a few suggestions for getting started.

safe space

Call to mind an image of yourself as a child of four or five. What would have made bedtime feel safe and cozy — or safer and cozier — for your childhood self? Now give your adult self that same sense of comfort. Wrap yourself in a soft blanket or, what the heck, choose a stuffed animal to bring with you to bed. Even if your childhood was happy and safe, it doesn't hurt to pamper yourself with an extra layer of comfort at night.

extra dark

Simply by picking up this book you have made a commitment to improving your relationship to sleep and dreams. So, reward yourself with a special treat. I recommend a nice bar of dark chocolate. Decadent though it sounds, dark chocolate is good medicine for those who crave comforting sleep. Dark (80 percent or greater) chocolate contains a healthy dose of magnesium, which supports our circadian rhythms, thus preparing the body for nighttime sleep. If you're sensitive to caffeine, which is also present in chocolate, be sure to enjoy your treat early in the day.

SO, LET'S GET STARTED. And what better place to begin than at the end — meaning at the end of day, as we prepare for sleep. After all, in Genesis, the world begins in darkness, and then God says, "Let there be light." In this book, too, we'll begin at night, and move through preparations for bedtime, sleep, and dreams. After all, we need to sleep in order to rest, refresh, and renew ourselves, so we can wake up well.

*There is a time
for many words,
a time for sleep
as well.*

HOMER, *THE ODYSSEY*

a good night's sleep

...

Who looks outside, dreams.
Who looks inside, awakes.

CARL JUNG

These days there's a lot of talk about "waking up." Self-help books (even this one) and motivational speakers rally us to wake up to one form of spiritual truth or another, or to enlightenment in general. And I think that's great.

But in our earnest haste to reach the peak of our potential, we tend to skip a few steps — or even an entire staircase. With apologies to all the Type A personalities out there who were hoping for a tidy to-do list for solving their sleep problems, decoding dreams, and scaling spiritual heights all at the same time, I have other plans for you. If you want to wake up — really wake up, that is — to your very best experience of life physically, emotionally, and spiritually, you first need a good night's rest.

›

After all, there's a reason we're programmed to sleep for a third of our lives. When we close our eyes at night, we fall into a cycle of sleep: light sleep followed by deep sleep, then active, dream-filled sleep. This cycle, which repeats several times during the night, is crucial to repairing, restoring, and recharging the body so we can get the most from our days.

In this section we'll look at the role sleep plays in our lives, touch on the science of sleep, and offer plenty of suggestions for approaching sleep mindfully so you can settle in for a sweet rest.

SLUMBER PAL

We spend nearly as much time sleeping as we do working — and in some cases more. We may even log more hours asleep than we do interacting with our loved ones. And yet, for the most part we take sleep for granted and know very little about it.

Take a few moments now to get to know your nightly companion, Sleep. Respond to the following imaginative prompts with your first thoughts, without censoring or judging yourself. Just have fun.

› *If Sleep were a person, its name would be* _____.

› *If I could talk to Sleep, I'd tell it* _____.

› *If I could ask one thing of Sleep, it would be* _____?

› *If Sleep could speak, it might tell me* _____.

› *And it might ask me* _____?

› *To continue to get to know Sleep better, I will* _____.

BED

I t's the home base we scramble to reach after a long day, and it's the place from which we begin again each morning. Bed is where we sleep and dream; throughout the ages it has also been where babies are birthed, and where we go to die. In bed we nestle and nest, cocoon and create new life. It's where we can create the conditions that help us wake with inspiration and innovative ideas.

Bed. The compact word is made up of a lowercase *b* and *d* facing each other like a matching headboard and footboard. Between them, a small *e* curls around itself like a baby asleep on a plump mattress. This single syllable has wide-ranging roots from many languages: from the Germanic *bhedh* or *bajam*, meaning "a place dug into the ground like a garden or grave" to the Greek *bothyros*, meaning "pit" — which perhaps takes its meaning from the animal's primal bed, a small crater dug into layers of leaves and dirt. In Old

English the word means "the bottom of the lake or sea." Indeed, in bed asleep we dive into the mysteries of consciousness, that ravine of memory and association as deep as the collective ground of human history, our human story.

Bed. Animals make theirs, too: roosting in rafters, nesting in branches, huddling in hay. Even at sea, dolphins doze in moonlit currents.

The bed, like the one bedded down in it, takes countless forms: trekkers stretch out on whisper-thin pads, the homeless find what comfort they can on park benches or in cardboard boxes sited on subway grates, and kings curtain themselves beneath canopies of sumptuous embroidery. Be it a humble pallet or an elaborately carved and crafted bedstead, it's where we spoon with our lovers and cuddle our babies. We share our covers with favorite pets, or lie down with only our dreams, while the planets spin and the stars shine.

Bed. Like the ground beneath our feet or the air we breathe, our bed is a constant source of support that we often take for granted. But it's likely the first of our possessions to be pushed through the doorway of a new home, dragged up the steps and dropped into place, while all of our other belongings pile in boxes in the center of some as-yet-unpainted room to be sorted out later.

They say home is where you hang your hat — but really it's where we make our bed that defines our digs and allows us to dig in and begin our lives anew each day.

• • • • • • • •

TUCK IN

Hygge (pronounced *hoo-ga*) is a Danish word that means "coziness," and evokes the scent of cinnamon, comfy wool socks in winter, and conversation with friends by candlelight. The Danish love for all things hygge is said to be one reason Denmark has been rated one of the happiest countries. At its heart, hygge is about appreciating the simple things and bringing more comfort into our lives. What better place to begin paying attention to everyday pleasures than the bedroom, where we tuck in for the night.

get comfortable

What comforts you? It could be a person, a pet, or a place, or even an activity, such as sewing or swimming. Make a list of things that bring you comfort (include scents, sounds, colors, or tastes) and refer to it again and again. Commit to bringing more comfort, in all its many forms, into your life. Then share some (in the form of kind words or gestures) with others whenever you can.

make your bed

Turn the first chore of the day into a gratitude practice. As you smooth out the sheets and shake the blankets back into place, focus your thoughts. Rather than let your mind wander aimlessly, anchor your attention to your breath. Notice the sensation of your hands as you fluff the pillows and tug the covers taut, and consciously consider all the ways this expansive piece of furniture adds to your life. It is the place where you sit and read, make love, sleep, and dream. Send some gratitude to your bed for all the ways it supports you, literally and figuratively, and for setting the stage for a safe and sound night of sleep.

it's not just what we do in bed that matters

Conventional wisdom for healthy sleep hygiene holds that the bed should be for making love and sleeping only. But just as important as what we do in bed are the thoughts we take with us when we go there. Make your bed a worry-free zone. Banish troubles from your mind by writing them in your journal, and close the covers on them before you turn off the lights.

• • • • • • • •

CREATE YOUR SLEEP SANCTUARY

We might close our eyes encircled in the arms of our beloved, but once we cross into sleep we are, in a very real sense, alone. That may be why we tend to lavish more of our decorative flourishes and housekeeping prowess on other rooms while leaving our beds unmade or heaping our clothes on a chair in the corner. We close the bedroom door, knowing that no one else will see that pocket of neglect anyway. But to reflect the value of sleep and dreams, the bedroom should be a haven of comfort and peace.

what's the message?

If there are phones, computers, or file folders from work dropped on the bureau in your bedroom, you are giving your subconscious the message that this is a place for doing, not relaxing. Clothes strewn about? What does that say about how you value your time in the bedroom? Look at your room anew and assess what messages it's sending to your subconscious about your attitude toward sleep. Remove or replace any items that don't support your intention to rest and relax in this space.

fluff it up

Now, turn your attention to the condition of your mattress and pillows. If they're worse for wear and no longer serve your goal of getting your best night's sleep, it may be time to replace them. Consider mattress toppers, buckwheat pillows, and other bed accessories that can help you settle in for a good rest. (Hint: don't be shy, survey your friends about what works for them. If someone sings the praises of their pillow, mattress, or topper, ask if you can take a nap at their place to see if their recommendations work for your body. Also, peek under the sheets and check out the make of mattresses that bring you comfort when you wake well rested at a hotel or inn while traveling.)

snuggle up

Cuddling boosts oxytocin, a hormone that makes you feel good, reduces stress and anxiety, and improves sleep. Touching in various forms, including holding hands, massage, and sex, encourages the body's production of oxytocin. If you sleep alone, you can also gain the benefits of the love hormone by petting your dog or cat, thinking about pleasurable experiences, or taking a warm bubble bath before bed.

sleep scents

The right aromas can support sound sleep. Use a diffuser in your bedroom with calming essential oils such as lavender, sandalwood, or pine, all of which invite relaxation. Or add a plant whose scent is known to soothe sleepy souls — such as jasmine, gardenia, or valerian — to the bedside table or nearby windowsill.

boring is better

Adrenaline-fueled adventure novels are best kept out of your bedroom. Instead, try soothing stories for your bedtime reads; those with endearing characters and pleasantly predictable plotlines will do just fine.

Lullaby
and good night,
with roses bedight
With lilies o'er spread
is baby's wee bed
Lay thee down now
and rest,
may thy slumber
be blessed

BRAHMS' LULLABY

LULLABY

Traditionally composed in the triple meter of ballads and waltzes, the lullaby's rhythm and melody evoke primal memories of the watery womb, the beating heart, and the bouncing knee. Add to that lyrics redolent with silvery moonbeams, roses, angels, twinkling stars, and mockingbirds, and you have the magic recipe that can sway even a stubbornly crying baby to sleep.

Except of course when the boughs break and babies tumble from cradles. Or when, as in some traditional sleep songs, lyrics lurch into tales of crying infants who are threatened with attacks by hungry hyenas or punishing wolves if they don't keep quiet and behave.

The stark contrasts between the nursery songs' rocking-chair comfort and cradle-crashing rhymes hint at our uneasy stance in the face of sleep. Throughout time and across cultures, lullabies simultaneously plead for safety and repose and call up stark reminders of the dangers that lurk in the cold, dark night.

The very word *lullaby* is a study in contrasts. The *lull* in *lullaby* whispers of the cushioned caress of our first in-utero sleep. But *lull* can also refer to that menacing stillness between stormy winds. And so the lullaby seems intent on reminding us that even the most restful of sleeps can be interrupted by a sudden night-shattering clang of fear, the thrumming threat of predators real or imagined, or ghouls and spirits who can't be kept out with even the strongest locks or the sturdiest doors.

Then there's that farewell note at the end of the word: *by*, as in goodbye. It's the false cheer of a jaunty "God be with you" — cold consolation to the traveler stepping over the threshold into the unknown.

These lullabies, whose lyrics were once carved into ancient clay and now populate playlists on our thoroughly modern devices, are sung in hushed whispers in the dark by the people who love us most. They acknowledge the mysteries and danger we confront when we lie down to sleep, but they also comfort us with golden strands of prayer, hope, and love. In this way, they have much to teach us about presence and courage in the face of fear. And so we ride their music, like magic carpets that carry us on their lightly hypnotic melodies across the chasm of night and into morning.

· · · · · · · ·

A LITTLE NIGHT MUSIC

Too often, rather than the sweet sounds of sleep songs, the brash tones of television voices fill our homes in the evening. Or maybe there is only the silent swiping of phone screens as we check status updates one last time before bed. Here are some ways to bring the music of lullabies back into your nighttime routine.

not just for babies

In addition to being an age-old sleep aid for infants, toddlers, and children, and a beautiful way for parents and babies to bond, lullabies have also been shown to reduce stress in the adults who sing them. Tonight, sing your children, your partner, or yourself to sleep. Find a sing-along CD or songbook to help you learn new songs or remind you of forgotten lyrics to old favorites.

don't just press play

Babies are known to sleep better and learn more when lullabies are sung to them by loving adults. So don't just press play — sing along.

sleep songs

Get the music started before you climb into bed. Create a bedtime playlist of soothing songs — traditional lullabies or not — to play while you go about your bedtime routine of brushing teeth and changing into pajamas. Let the sweet songs encourage the adults and children in your household to get delightfully sleepy as bedtime approaches.

sacred syllables

Various spiritual traditions offer chants or mantras to help people sleep. One Sanskrit mantra that is easy to remember, and which can calm and balance the mind for sleep, is *sa ta na ma*. These sounds mean "birth, life, death, and rebirth" and are said to help wake us to our divine nature. Sing these syllables to yourself before bed and feel your mind and body settle down for sleep. (To become familiar with the rhythm and melody of the chant, ask a yoga teacher or search for the chant online.)

All people are children
when they sleep.
There's no war
in them then.

ROLF JACOBSEN, "WHEN THEY SLEEP"

GETTING
SLEEPY

I t seems counterintuitive, and counter even to our species' primary task of survival: each night we lie down, defenseless, eyes closed, senses dulled. Our faculties for rational decision-making are tamped down. We do this not for a few brief moments   fingers crossed that our vulnerability won't be recognized or exploited — but for hours, the length of a complete nine-to-five workday, in fact. Risky though it is from an evolutionary point of view, sleep is vital to our physical, mental, and emotional health and well-being. We need it and crave it in the same way we need and crave food or water. If we deny ourselves sleep, our bodies will steal it from us whenever possible, whether it's when we sit down to watch TV, settle on the sofa with a novel propped on our knees, or, in extreme cases, when we drive through the night despite our inner cries for rest.

Some people can't wait to slip into bed at the end of the day, while others resist turning in and turning out the lights. Your early experiences with nighttime likely color your attitudes toward sleep today. But by making new decisions and updating your evening habits you can cozy up and experience a more enjoyable bedtime.

. . . .

EIGHT FOR EIGHT

Whether your ideal is to get six or eight hours of shut-eye each night, simple changes in routine have been proven to be as effective as medication for getting a good night's rest. Here are eight elements to enhance the quality of your sleep, naturally:

1. back into bedtime

To eat mindfully, we leave the table before we are overly full. To sleep mindfully, go to bed before you are maxed out with exhaustion. This can be difficult with so many activities and responsibilities competing for your time. But it's also the most important step. So, work backward when you plan your day, and build in a solid hour to wind down so you can climb into bed before you are beat.

SNOOZE REPORT

Reflect on your relationship with sleep by responding to these prompts in your journal. Write the first things that come to mind, spending just a few minutes on each question. Your answers might surprise you!

If I valued sleep more . . .

If I could change one thing about my experience of sleep, it would be . . .

2. commit to it

Spontaneity is great, but when it comes to sleep, sticking to a schedule works best. Make a commitment to go to bed at about the same time each night. Then, mark your calendar with a gold star or silly sticker for every night you succeed in tucking in on time. When you succeed for a whole week, treat yourself to something special that affirms your dedication to better sleep, such as a luxurious evening bubble bath, a soothing CD, or a scented eye pillow.

3. stretch before bed

Prepare the body for sleep with a few stretches or yoga poses that help soothe anxiety and still the mind: cat/cow, downward-facing dog, forward fold, and legs up the wall poses are all good options. (If you aren't familiar with these poses, you can find good instructions on yoga websites or consider taking a beginner's yoga class.)

4. mind your routines

Bring mindful attention to nighttime routines to prepare for a good night's sleep. For example, as you wash your face and brush your teeth, you might imagine that you are washing away any worries, regrets, or plans for tomorrow. Let any thoughts from your busy mind swirl down the drain with the soapy water as you exhale deeply and relax.

5. feed your spirit

Evening is a time to calm your energy, so watch what you ingest, both mentally and physically. Restrict your intake of news to daylight hours if possible, and focus on reading, doing, or watching things that encourage feelings of calm and well-being at night. What you eat after the sun goes down matters, too. Eat as little as possible in the three hours before bed, but if you need a snack, choose a slice of whole-grain toast, a small bowl of oatmeal sprinkled with slivered almonds, or a handful of cherries — which contain sleep-friendly doses of melatonin, magnesium, and tryptophan.

6. hit the cushion (before your head hits the pillow)

Meditating in the evening between dinner and bedtime calms the mind for sleep. Instructions for several meditations will be offered throughout this book (or if you already have a meditation practice that works for you, use that). Just 10 to 20 minutes will do.

7. divine mind

As you enter sleep, you might be heading toward anything from a peaceful night to scary dreams. You could be blessed with deep rest or hours of anxious thoughts and tossing and turning. So move through this transition consciously. Say a prayer, or set an intention to connect with the spirit of goodness, love, or peace just before you turn out the light.

8. gratitude for a good night

Studies show that people who go to bed grateful tend to sleep and dream better. As you drift into sleep, mentally review what you are thankful for, or mentally replay any beautiful or loving moments from your day.

*Early to bed and early to rise, makes
a man healthy, wealthy, and wise.*

BENJAMIN FRANKLIN

IT'S GOOD FOR YOU, AND IT FEELS GOOD, TOO

Doctors, scientists, lifestyle gurus, and talk-show hosts have been touting the benefits of getting enough exercise for decades. Now, the new trending topic is sleep. If you've been paying even the least bit of attention to the lifestyle pages of your favorite magazine or health blogs, you can probably reel off the benefits of getting enough sleep, well, in your sleep. As with a daily exercise regimen, regularly getting a good night's sleep reduces stress, boosts your mood, helps manage weight, repairs memory, and even makes our skin and hair shine.

And so doctors write prescriptions for sleep medications, and life coaches talk about proper sleep hygiene, all of which can make going to bed feel a bit clinical. We've wandered from the comfort of lullabies, teddy bears, and rocking chairs into a muddled morass of worry, calculation, and medical evaluation as we approach bedtime. Sadly, sleep has become one more thing to stress out about.

But there is another way. Rather than medicalizing sleep, we can approach it with loving attention and caring intention.

BEDTIME CHECKUP

Check in with yourself to see how you are thinking and talking about sleep. Here are a few subtle, but helpful, points to consider.

expect the best

If sleep often eludes you, you might understandably have slipped into negative thinking patterns around it. Our thoughts cue our subconscious mind, and we can inadvertently program ourselves for a fitful night. But you can reprogram yourself, too. Think about the kind of sleep you want to experience, and write it down in the form of an affirmative statement in the present tense such as, "I let go, relax, and welcome satisfying, sound sleep." Repeat your affirmation to yourself several times before bed or whenever you think about sleep.

word power

A simple goodnight kiss, along with a sweet bedtime wish, does wonders for creating a cozy mood for sleep. Wish your family members good and pleasant dreams before bed . . . and wish the same for yourself. If you live alone, send good sleep wishes out to your friends and loved ones, wherever they are.

out of your head

Electronic devices and pints of ice cream are among the things you know you shouldn't bring to bed with you if you want a good night's sleep. But the number-one sleep stealer is in your head. Bringing to bed your negative thoughts, problems, plans, and regrets crushes your chances of getting much-needed rest. To get out of your head, give yourself a soothing foot rub before bed. Use warm massage oil (organic sesame oil is a good choice) or relaxing rose-scented moisturizing cream. Then slip on some cozy socks and let your happy feet guide you into sleep.

head-to-toe flow

With this simple relaxation technique you will bring your attention to each of your body's energy centers, or chakras, to help ease you into sleep.

1. Begin by lying on your back in bed and settling into stillness by taking a few slow, conscious breaths.

2. Now place the palms of both of your hands on the crown of your head, and take three slow and conscious breaths while you focus your relaxed attention on the top of your head.

3. Leaving your left hand on the crown of your head, move your right hand to your forehead, with fingertips resting on the spot between your eyebrows, and again take three slow, easy breaths. Continue by moving the right hand down to each position as described in the following steps (next page), while leaving your left hand on the crown of your head.

4. Gently place your right hand on your throat, and take three slow, conscious breaths here.

5. Next, move your hand to your heart center, and take three more breaths here.

6. Now move your hand to your solar plexus, in the space just below where your two bottom ribs meet, and take three breaths here.

7. Next, move your hand to your abdomen, just below your navel, and take three breaths here.

8. Then place your hand on your pubic bone, and again take three slow, easy breaths here.

9. Finally, move your left hand to meet your right hand, and place both palms facing down in the space between your hipbones and the top of your pubic bone, with fingertips forming a downward-facing V. Settle here for three more breaths.

10. When you are ready, move into a comfortable sleeping position, and allow yourself to let go and drift into deep rest.

CYCLES OR STAGES

the geometry of sleep

S cientists often speak of sleep in terms of stages. But I prefer to speak of sleep cycles. That's because "stages," like steps, are raised and require effort to climb. Cycles, on the other hand, bring to mind things that flow effortlessly, with no endpoint to strive toward. This is a more soothing — and more accurate — image for the process of moving from sleep to dreams to waking, then returning again to sleep to begin again.

This cycle is marked by the release of various neurochemicals that prompt movement between light sleep, deep and deeper sleep, and dreams. But the wheel doesn't stop turning there. During the day, our brain chemistry adjusts, too, as we move from focused attention to relaxed attention, daydreaming, or mind-wandering.

Imagining consciousness as flowing between various states of brain activity can help us integrate sleep more seamlessly into our lives rather than banish it to the basement of our priority list, as we too often do.

. . . .

ROUNDING OUT THE DAY

It pays to notice the subtle changes our bodies and minds cycle through each day so we can get in sync with our natural rhythms. Here are some ways to get started.

attention span

You've heard about sleep stages, but our consciousness is shifting all day long. Every 90 minutes or so our brains cycle through different types of focus. Take advantage of this cycle by doing your work or tasks in 90-minute segments, allowing your brain to rest for several minutes between each one. Frequent breaks are said to improve productivity.

clock watch

Digital readouts on clocks, watches, and phones reinforce the sense that time is marching forward in a linear column of minutes and hours. A round-faced clock, whose hands turn in sleepy circles around its face, can remind us of the cyclical nature of wake, sleep, and dreams, and invite you to take a more relaxed view of time. Consider replacing your bedroom clock with one that has a friendly, round design.

sunrise, sunset

Celebrate the subtle shifts between night and day, and day and night, by watching a sunrise or sunset. When you do, pay attention: can you see the moment when dusk turns to night or dawn to morning?

YOUR LAPTOP IS NOT A TEDDY BEAR

It seems we've traded in our teddy bears for high-tech gizmos. According to a poll by the National Sleep Foundation, 9 out of 10 Americans say they use an electronic device (TV, cell phone, computer) in the hour before bed, and many report bringing laptops, tablets, and phones into bed with them. But if we don't put our devices to sleep, we're not likely to get much shut-eye either. The screens we stare into emit an electronic glow that interferes with melatonin production, inhibiting our natural rhythms of sleep and waking. What's more, depending on what we're doing online (answering emails, posting on social media, playing games), we're also revving up the brain when we should be slowing down. In the process, stress hormones, such as cortisol, are released, and the Land of Nod recedes into the distance.

TAMING TECHNOLOGY FOR BETTER SLEEP

In the best-case scenario, we should declare our bedrooms tech-free zones and turn off all electronics a half hour or more before heading to bed. But if that seems like too large a leap to take all at once, we can take small but effective steps to balance the benefits of technology with our need for a good night's sleep.

alert yourself

Program an alert on your phone to signal when it's time to power down and begin your bedtime routine. When the alarm sounds, turn off electronic devices, and stop any activities that require mental or physical effort.

bye-bye blue light

Adjust your phone, tablet, or laptop's screen settings to filter out the attention-boosting blue light, which disturbs natural circadian rhythms, or use the backlight option. You can use an app with a red filter, program your devices to do this for you automatically, or do it manually when the sun sets.

no-phone zone

Minimize the use of phones and other electronics by covering unused outlets with plug protectors (sold as child-safety products) to discourage yourself from charging electronics in the bedroom. Then, when your phone or laptop runs low on batteries, you'll be less inclined to give it more juice, and more inclined to settle down and recharge your own batteries.

the passive choice

Not all electronics are created equal when it comes to interfering with sleep. More passive technologies, like television, cause less sleep interference than ones we engage with more actively, such as computer games or online chatting.

new life for dead phones

Use outdated phones that are no longer connected to cellular services as alarm clocks, bedside MP3 players, and voice recorders for recording dreams. That way you can enjoy these features without having your sleep interrupted by incoming calls or messages — and avoid the temptation to read email, check social media, or surf the Web.

*Taking one of the
stones there, he put it
under his head and lay
down to sleep.*

GENESIS 28:11

PILLOW

S leep may give us time to rest our bodies, but really it is the playground for the mind. In fact, our brain is as active during dreams as it is when awake. It makes sense then that we cushion our head in comfort, enthroning it for the night.

Stuffed with feathers or foam, pillows are billowy clouds of comfort, but soft, fluffy pillows are a relatively modern invention. In ancient times (dating back to about 7000 BCE) Egyptians used stones for pillows. Clearly comfort was not the goal. Instead the stone pillows were used to elevate the head to keep insects from crawling in and out of the sleeper's nose, mouth, and ears. In

Asia, where pillows were also once made of hard materials like wood, stone, or porcelain, people believed their pillows could infuse the brain with the material's attributes. For example, a pillow of jade was believed to boost the intellect. Other types of pillow were said to have the power to cure headaches or depression.

Soft pillows stuffed with feathers, reeds, or straw and encased in embroidered fabrics were a later innovation, credited to the ancient Greeks and Romans. These luxurious headrests were rare, expensive, and often reserved for kings and queens. Then the Industrial Revolution made textiles more accessible to common people. But in some times and places, pillows were scoffed at as a sign of weakness. In Tudor England, for example, only women giving birth were allowed the luxury of using a pillow.

Whether your bed is topped with pillows that are stuffed with synthetic fibers, foam, flaxseed, or down, take a moment tonight to whisper a small prayer of gratitude for having a comfortable place on which to rest your sleepy head.

• • • • • • • •

THE SOFT SPOT

What if we were to bring the same soulful intention to our time on the pillow in bed as we might to the meditation cushion or the yoga mat? Here are some ways your pillow can help inspire sweet sleep and satisfying dreams.

sleep stone

Use your pillow as a plush touchstone. Each time your head lands on it, take a moment to acknowledge your intention for a good night's rest and helpful dreams.

pillow art

Shop for a beautiful pillowcase that reflects your commitment to honoring sleep and inviting good dreams. Or purchase some fabric and sew your own. If you're feeling extra crafty, you can even use fabric markers or embroidery thread to decorate a plain or patterned pillowcase.

beneath your pillow

Children tuck their baby teeth beneath their pillows for the tooth fairy, and in some cultures mothers slip cloves of garlic under a sick child's pillow for healing. An amethyst placed under the pillow is said to ease insomnia and bring soothing dreams. Consider placing a small item beneath your pillow to remind you of your intentions for enjoying a sound sleep.

• • • • • • • •

DREAM SCENTS

Dream pillows are sachets filled with herbs that are said to stimulate dreams, improve dream recall, or help you relax into deep sleep. These herb-filled pouches can be tucked into your pillowcase or slipped beneath your pillow. Make or buy a dream pillow with herbs that support your desire for a good night's sleep and dreams. Here are some traditional dream pillow herbs along with their properties for promoting sleep and dreams:

ANGELICA • Dreams and visions

BAY LAUREL • Inspiration

HOPS • Healing, rest

JASMINE • Psychic dreams, relieves depression

LAVENDER • Relaxation, deep sleep

MARJORAM • Relieves depression

MUGWORT • Visions and prophetic dreams

ROSE PETALS • Prophetic dreams

VALERIAN • Rest and relaxation

Sleep is the best meditation.

DALAI LAMA

OMS FOR Z'S

lessons from yoga and meditation

Both yoga and meditation help people develop their ability to stay conscious and awake to their thoughts and feelings and to live each moment with intention. And yet, when it comes to sleep and dreaming, even those who are dedicated practitioners often abandon what they've learned on the yoga mat or meditation cushion and instead collapse onto the mattress, exhausted, leaving their minds free to wander aimlessly through dreams till morning.

In the pages that follow, we'll offer suggestions for bringing increased calm and clarity to sleep and dreams by bringing some lessons from the mat and cushion to the bed and pillow.

• • • • • • • •

GET SETTLED

You might feel so tired some nights that you just want to drop into bed. But pausing to more consciously position yourself for sleep (both physically and mentally) can make all the difference.

posture

Yoga teaches us to properly align our bodies to support increased flexibility and strength. Posture counts when it comes to sleep, too. Do a body scan in bed, taking a mental inventory of your entire body from your scalp to your toes to find any areas of discomfort or constriction. Reposition yourself or use an extra pillow to support your hip, shoulder, or leg until you find a supportive posture for sleep.

notice the moment

Watch your thoughts as you lie in bed. See if you can be present enough to notice the moment you cross the threshold from waking to sleep. But don't be discouraged if you can't. This is a practice whose reward is in the attempt; even meditation masters rarely meet this goal.

. . . .

BREATHING TOWARD INNER HARMONY

Relax in bed? Let go of worries? Sounds good, but how do you do it? The easiest way is to focus on your breathing, which simultaneously calms your nervous system and slows your thoughts. That's why simple yogic breathing techniques can soothe you into sleep. This yogic breathing exercise, or *pranayama*, is easy to learn and helps balance and quiet the mind for sleep.

1. With the palm of your right hand facing you, fold down the pointer and middle finger, keeping the other fingers extended.

2. Close your right nostril with your right thumb and inhale slowly and gently through the left nostril.

3. Lightly close the left nostril with your ring finger and little finger so both nostrils are held closed for a brief pause.

4. Open your right nostril and exhale slowly through the right; then inhale slowly on the same side.

5. Gently close the right nostril with your right thumb, and pause for just a moment as you hold both nostrils closed again.

6. Open your left nostril and exhale slowly; then inhale slowly on the same side.

7. Repeat the cycle several times before sleep.

8. On each exhalation let go of worries or concerns from the day. With each inhalation, breathe in peace and contentment.

FROM A TO Z'S . . .

Here is another way to calm the mind and prepare for sleep. Before bed, take five minutes to create your "A List." Focus on these five areas (each beginning with the letter *A*), and in your journal, reflect briefly on each one.

ADORATION. Where have I felt and expressed my love today? Have I told family members how much I appreciate them? Today, have I felt reverence or awe for some ordinary delight (by taking a moment to smile at the sparkle of falling snow, or pausing to pet the cat who lounges atop a shelf at my favorite bookstore)?

ATONEMENT. Where did I fall short today? Do I owe anyone an apology? Do I need to forgive myself for something?

APPRECIATION. Did I feel gratitude and show appreciation today? Did I thank the person who held the door for me as I rushed about on my errands today? Did I offer a word of praise to a coworker? What do I feel grateful for right now?

ANTICIPATION. What am I looking forward to doing or experiencing tomorrow? It may be as simple as that first cup of coffee or as special as dinner with a dear friend. Whatever it is, savor the feeling of looking ahead with joy.

ASK FOR IT. Bedtime is the ideal time to pose a question to your wisest self, God, the divine, the universe, or whatever you call that benevolent force that brings you comfort. Ask for guidance about a problem or insight into a pressing issue, or simply request a restful night of sleep. Write your question in your journal, and watch for an answer in your dreams or in the thoughts that come to you when you wake in the morning.

WHEN SLEEP WON'T COME

It's four in the morning, and you're wide awake. Anxiety wraps itself tightly around your chest, and your head is awash in worries. And now you're also worrying about not getting enough sleep. You count the hours until your alarm will ring, add up the hours you've slept so far, subtract from eight, and grow angry at the impossibility of any of this adding up to a good night's sleep. You try to march your mind back into sleepiness by counting backwards or trying to remember the names of everyone in your first-grade class — all in a desperate attempt to nod off.

But this early morning period of wakefulness, so dreaded by insomniacs, is by contrast courted by meditation masters, monks, and mystics. Intentionally waking before dawn, they meditate in the quiet and stillness of these early hours.

Meanwhile, most of us can't seem to find time to meditate during the busy day. Even 20 minutes seems like too much when you have work, family responsibilities, a home to care for, and social engagements. You may have social media pages to maintain and keep up with, as well as streaming music and television series competing for your attention. But at four o'clock in the morning there's nothing on the calendar, no phones ringing, and the laptop is sleeping — even if you aren't. So why not use this time to meditate? (See page 53 for a good method for nighttime meditation.)

After all, meditation is a proven natural and effective antidote to insomnia. Plus, it's better to feel a little holy rather than wholly frustrated when you're up, especially if your loved one snores serenely nearby.

You need not follow rigid rules for a middle-of-the-night meditation. You don't even need to leave your bed. Unlike in formal meditation, when it's considered bad form and a sign of flagging focus to doze off, when you meditate on the mattress for relaxation, falling asleep is an added bonus. Sure, the meditation practice was cut short, but then again you got some much-needed sleep. Plus, if you do slip into sleep directly from meditation, you're more likely to experience clear and, sometimes, even lucid or luminous dreams.

Then again, if you don't fall asleep, you've still managed to meditate for 45 minutes to an hour, thus achieving an equally beneficial outcome — you've reaped the rewards of a successful meditation session, which include reduced stress, improved heart health, and a boost to your mood. And since brain scans of people in deep meditation resemble those of people in deep sleep, you're likely to start the day feeling rested, too.

• • • • • • • • •

BEDITATE

Effort is the enemy of sleep. So, stop trying so hard to catch some z's. Instead, bring the wisdom of meditation as well as simple relaxation techniques to bed with you.

count breaths, not thoughts

The late-night brain is notably low on serotonin and other neurochemicals that help boost our mood by day. Therefore, nighttime — when our minds are likely to devolve into pessimism and negative thinking — is no time to ponder problems. Instead, puzzle over something neutral. Numbers, rather than words, work best for midnight meditations. Count backward by threes from 300 (i.e., 300, 297, 294). Or count your breaths one by one, starting at 10 and working backward. When you get to 1, start at 10 again, repeating the process until you doze off. Bring your full attention to each number as you count down, leaving no room in your mind for worrisome thoughts.

on the pillow

You can sit up in bed and meditate or lie on your back with your arms at your sides (think *savasana*, or relaxation pose, from yoga class). You may prefer to rest the palms of your hands on your abdomen, which can help you feel calm.

hit play

Keep an MP3 or CD player loaded with ready-to-play guided meditations by your bed. When you can't sleep, just press play, listen, and relax. (To find some good recorded meditations, you can do an Internet search, browse your local bookstore, or ask a yoga or meditation teacher for suggestions.)

• • • • • • • •

PRODUCTIVE REST

Happily, there is a way to get some deep rest, even if you can't sleep. The practice of yoga nidra, or yogic sleep, is a form of meditation that helps you feel refreshed and at ease, and may even make you feel as if you've slept deeply. Yoga nidra is also said to reduce tension, ease anxiety, and support and strengthen the immune system.

The practice, which involves bringing attention systematically to each part of the body, is simple and easy. Done during the day, yoga nidra allows you to enter a state close to that of dreamless sleep while remaining awake and aware. At night, for help sleeping, you can follow the same process but without the intention to remain awake.

yoga nidra basics

To practice yoga nidra, you will scan your body in a slow, methodical, thorough way, resting your full and relaxed attention on each part of your body for the length of a breath or two. Although you will feel very relaxed during this process, try to stay aware and awake. But don't worry if you fall asleep or if you don't follow the instructions precisely. These are general guidelines, and there are many variations to this practice. However, if you are practicing yoga nidra during the day and want to be sure you don't fall asleep, set an alarm to signal the end of your practice, just in case.

I recommend giving yourself 20 to 40 minutes for this leisurely exercise. You can find recordings online or on CD that will guide you through yoga nidra, or follow the basic steps listed at right.

1. Lie on your back on a yoga mat on the floor or on another soft yet supported surface. Cover yourself with a sheet or blanket to stay comfortably warm and relaxed.

2. Close your eyes and allow your arms and legs to open at a slight angle so they are not touching the body or each other, as in savasana.

3. Spend a minute or two observing the breath rise and fall in your belly, allowing your breath to slow down and lengthen as your thoughts, too, begin to slow.

4. Rest your attention on your mouth, including lips, tongue, gums, and jaw. Observe each part of the mouth for the length of a breath or two.

5. Continue to move your relaxed, nonjudgmental, curious attention methodically along your body, resting your awareness on each part:

   - Your head, including ears, nose, eyes, forehead, scalp, neck, and throat, inside and outside

   - Your arms, one at a time, including the shoulder, upper arm, elbow, lower arm, wrist, palm of the hand, and each finger, one by one

   - Your torso, front and back, including your upper chest, solar plexus, belly, and abdomen

   - Your pelvis, hips, sacrum, base of the spine, and genitals

   - Your legs, including the upper leg, lower leg, ankles, top of the foot, bottom of the foot, and each toe, one by one

6. When you have completed your scan, bring your attention back to the room you are in, notice the sounds, the sensations on your skin, and the weight of your body resting on the mat or other surface.

7. Turn on your side and rest for a few more breaths. When you are ready, gradually move to a seated position. Take your time getting up.

If we sit with an increasing
stillness of the body,
and attune our mind
to the sky or to the ocean
or to the myriad stars at night,
or any other indicators of vastness,
the mind gradually stills
and the heart is filled
with quiet joy.

RAVI RAVINDRA

DARKNESS, SILENCE, AND STILLNESS, OH MY!

We live in a world of pulsing, glowing, flashing lights, where we have all but banished darkness and drowned silence in a stream of music and chatter that we've literally wired into our ears.

In the checkout line at the supermarket, in the waiting room at the dentist's or doctor's office, or even driving in your car, notice that it doesn't take more than a minute or two before you or someone around you begins to tap their toe, jiggle their knee, or thumb their phone's screen. It is rare to find a person these days who is truly comfortable in stillness. And then we scratch our heads and ask why it's so hard to quiet our thoughts, relax, and drift into sleep.

Ironically, the very things we need most to settle in and fall asleep are the things we tend to resist and fear: darkness, stillness, and a silent surrender to our inner world. It's time to reclaim these precious resources in any way we can.

• • • • • • • •

BE STILL

In order to enter into sleep, we have to stop fidgeting, stop doing, and settle down. With a little practice, we can all learn the art of being — instead of always doing.

spend some time

Take a few moments each day to observe something that's still: a tree, a mountain, or a child in deep sleep. Try to locate that feeling of calm somewhere inside yourself.

soften into the stillness inside

Next time you habitually reach for something to read, do, watch, or eat when you could instead just sink into stillness, observe how you are feeling inside. You may notice that you are experiencing discomfort, disappointment, mild anxiety, fear, or restlessness. Try to soften toward your feelings and accept them rather than distract yourself from them. Observe your body and your thoughts without trying to change anything. Can you notice — and accept — the stillness deep inside you?

find your center

Get comfortable, take a few cleansing breaths, and bring your attention to your solar plexus, the spot just below where your bottom ribs meet. Keeping your attention here, tune into the gentle rhythms of your breath. Can you find the stillness just behind that quiet movement? Keep trying. Don't worry if you can't locate it. Even the search for stillness within will help you get closer to it.

• • • • • • • • •

NIGHT LIGHT

It's natural to be drawn to things that are light, happy, and positive, but if we completely reject, repress, or bury anything that has to do with darkness and night we get into trouble. Darkness is not an enemy to be conquered or even something to be avoided. Rather, in the unlit spaces of our lives we find the fertile ground of creativity and imagination. You might even find that darkness can teach you to see what your eyes cannot. So, instead of resisting the transition from light into dark or rushing through it, impatient for the light of dawn, try instead to befriend the night.

pause, then flip

Each time you reach to flip on a light switch, pause, and first consider the darkness. Take a moment to check in with your inner darkness — your emotions and thoughts — before turning on the light.

You, darkness,
of whom I am born —
I love you more than the flame
that limits the world
to the circle it illumines.

RAINER MARIA RILKE

black gold

Consider the riches of dark fertile soil, black compost, the miraculous darkness of the womb that brings forth life, the beauty of onyx or obsidian, or the diamond glittering deep in the blackness of the mine. Make a list of the valuable things (literally and metaphorically speaking) that belong to — or come from — the dark.

night beauty

Whether at the drafting table, potter's wheel, the canvas, or the keyboard, the artist first closes her eyes in order to see something that has not yet come into existence. Only after tapping into the darkness of the unseen, the unwritten, or the unknown can she create something new. Make a collage or painting using predominantly dark colors or images. Celebrate the beauty in the dark.

bedroom blackout

We sleep better in the dark, so take steps to block out unnecessary light:

- To create complete darkness, remove, or at least cover, any electronic equipment in your bedroom that has glowing LED displays or lights.

- Hang curtains or shades to block the light shining through bedroom windows.

- Wear a sleep mask. As a bonus, the gentle pressure on your eyes will help still your eyeballs, which helps still your thoughts — so you can settle into peaceful darkness and get a good night's rest.

• • • • • • • •

THE PEACE IN QUIET

We claim to cherish it, but we resist silence at every turn. We rush to fill the gaps in conversation; we turn on the television even though we're not listening; and we crank the car stereo as soon as we turn on the ignition. Even when we do achieve something close to silence, we may not be satisfied. That's because what we really crave is not so much the absence of noise but a particular quality of quiet. We need the peace of inner acceptance and the ability to be still and quiet inside even in the presence of the screech of a far-off siren or the chatter in a crowded café. Here are some ways to find the quiet — inside and out — that we need in order to relax, rest deeply, and sleep.

the silent treatment

During the day, practice listening to the silences between sounds. Listen for the space between words during a conversation. Create a space the length of one exhalation between when your friend stops talking and when you respond. When you are by yourself and when you are meditating, listen for the gaps between your thoughts. Can you extend those silences and make them just a little longer?

quiet time

Choose 20 minutes or more each day to enjoy silence. Turn off the radio and television or anything with a volume control on it, and don't talk or take phone calls during this time. You can do this alone or with a family member or friend. Observe how you feel within silence.

the quietest sound

Try this meditation while sitting up or lying in bed as you wait for sleep to come.

1. Slow and relax your breathing for three to five breaths as you do a quick body scan to find any areas of discomfort. Let go of any tension with the exhalation.

2. Now focus on the sounds in your environment. Simply notice them without judgment and without naming or labeling them. If any thoughts come to mind let them drift past, and return your focus to the sounds around you.

3. For the next two or three breaths, choose one sound to focus on. Without judgment, without wishing it were different, and without labeling it, simply notice the sound.

4. Now, notice a quieter sound, and observe it in the same way for two or three more breaths.

5. Keep listening for progressively quieter sounds. Can you hear the beating of your own heart? The gentle pulses of air moving through your lungs, lifting your diaphragm, filling and emptying in your belly? Can you hear the silence deep in the center of your being? Keep listening.

hush

Take stock of your sleeping environment and reduce or eliminate sounds that might disturb your sleep, if possible.

- Fix a leaking faucet, or oil the hinges on a creaking door. If necessary, talk to your bed partner about strategies for treating snoring.

- Use an electric fan or noise machine to neutralize distracting or annoying sounds in your environment and create the peace needed to sleep.

- Set a noise curfew with family members or housemates. Restrict the use of phones and televisions after that time, unless they're enjoyed with earphones or headphones.

- To manage sounds you can't eliminate or reduce, purchase a pair of foam earplugs that will dull some of the sounds in your environment. Keep them close to your bed in easy reach so you'll have them when needed.

God is the friend
of silence.

MOTHER THERESA

sweet
dreams

...

*Sometimes dreams are wiser
than waking.*

BLACK ELK

Some people act as though paying attention to dreams is some far-out or esoteric activity, but there is nothing more natural than dreaming. Everybody does it! The barista who handed you your chai latte this morning dreams, and so does the person who cut you off in traffic. Your best friend dreams, and so does your best friend's dog. Even babies in utero dream.

The earliest records of human history, including sacred texts from cultures around the world, feature reports of dreams. Some say that Paleolithic cave paintings contained depictions of dreams.

>

What's more, many inventions and innovations came to us courtesy of dreams, including the periodic table and the sewing machine. If Albert Einstein hadn't taken his dreams seriously, we would not have had the theory of relativity, and if Stephenie Meyer didn't write hers down, she may have forgotten the idea for her first *Twilight* novel, which came to her in a dream.

Dreams really do matter. Whether you remember them or not, you dream several times each night, and the average person will have had some 200,000 dreams by the time he turns 80. And that's a good thing, because dreams offer insight, guidance, wisdom — and some truly magnificent new ideas.

But somehow we've been duped into believing that you need a psychology degree, a high-paid analyst, or at the very least a pile of dream dictionaries to understand something that is as natural to us as breathing. These are *your* dreams. They are the cumulative creative musings of your inner poet wooing you with sweet somethings. They are made of your unique memories and associations, and they come exclusively to you personally, special delivery, express mail, every night. Because they are speaking the language of your private hopes and fears, you don't need any special gifts to interpret them.

Another myth is that dreams merely happen *to* us, and require no attention on our part. But we can all benefit by becoming more mindful of our dreams, just as we benefit by being mindful about our thoughts. The first step is to be aware that we have dreams every night — whether we recall them or not — and to start to value them.

Beyond that, we can write our dreams down and study them for the meaning and messages they contain. We can learn to improve dream recall, and even to improve our ability to be more clear and conscious within our dreams, and to invite our dreams to help us with specific issues.

In this section we'll look at dreams from various angles and help you become a more active, engaged — and mindful — dreamer.

DREAM REFLECTIONS

Too few of us pay careful attention to our dreams. Let's start to change that now. In your journal, answer these questions about your relationship to your dreams:

› Do you remember your dreams daily? Occasionally? Just once in a blue moon?

› Do you dream in color? Have you heard music, tasted something, pinched yourself, or experienced smell in your dreams?

› What's the earliest dream you remember? What's the strangest dream you've ever had? The scariest? The best?

› Have you had recurring dreams?

› Have you ever known you were dreaming while you were dreaming?

› Have you ever had a dream that came true? Tell about it.

› Where do you think dreams come from? What have you been told by your parents or grandparents about dreams and why we have them? What do you believe?

Let it be.

THE BEATLES

A DREAM DEFINED

W hile I look forward each night to climbing into bed to see what my dreams have in store for me, many other people face their dreams with indifference or even dread. Either they are afraid of having nightmares or, more commonly, they find dreams so mystifying, confusing, and seemingly nonsensical that they shrug them off as reflexively as they wipe sleep from their eyes each morning.

And that's understandable. Dreams are difficult to pin down. What exactly are they, anyway? Where do they come from? Why do we have them at all? Dreams inspire questions but elude answers. Don't expect the dictionary to be of much help, either. Science reduces them to a series of largely random neurochemical interactions. But try as anyone might to box dreams into tidy categories, nothing can quite capture their vivid intensity or the way they can by turns entrance, captivate, frustrate, illuminate, terrify, and confound us. Dreams clothed in image and emotion defy easy description. And holding on to them can be like trying to catch a fish with only bare hands. They are weightless but weighty. They can't be measured, but some can't be shaken off.

They can creep up in the dark and give chase, give us pause, or give fright and leave many dreamers disillusioned, perplexed, or peeved.

Though many people don't realize it, the word *dream* itself has shadowy origins. Like the dream that we look to for meaning, so too the etymology of the word leads us on a labyrinthine and ultimately enlightening journey. The Sanskrit root *druh* means "to seek harm or to injure," and the Proto-Germanic *drachmas* means "deception, illusion, or phantasm." Look to the Old Norse and you'll find another fraught linguistic ancestor meaning "a ghost or apparition" — not exactly something you want to welcome into your bedroom at night with the lights out.

Square all of this with *dream*'s alternative lineage, if you can: The Old English or Old Saxon root *drom*, which may have grown up to become *dream*, is the distant relative of words like *joy*, *mirth*, and *merriment*.

So, like dreams themselves, the word contains curled within itself whispers of both the fear and celebration, the dread and bliss that we encounter when we encounter our dreams. But the more joyful branch of the etymological tree is where my relationship to dreams has blossomed. Having my dreams as companions, teachers, gurus, and guides has enriched my life. Sure, they sometimes wake me up frightened — but my dreams can also send me into laughter or spark a longing to stay in the beauty they conjure for just a little while longer.

• • • • • • • •

THE NO-SWEAT SCHOOL OF DREAMWORK

A lot of dreamwork books encourage you to "mine" your dreams for meaning, but that word conjures up images of coal dust and pick axes. Instead, have fun. Enjoy the imagery and intelligence in your dreams. Laugh at the puns they deliver. Put your feet up, place a paper umbrella in your drink, and relax that furrow in your brow. Consider these no-sweat approaches to working with your dreams instead.

the experience is enough

Before you rush to analyze a dream, first enjoy what your dreaming mind has delivered to you. Each dream is like a bird's nest woven of whimsical bits of memory, imagination, hope, and fear. Reflect on what your dream comprises: What aspects of your life are represented? Which of your life phases do the people and places in your dream remind you of? What colors appear in your dreams, and how do they make you feel? Then take a moment to be grateful for this gift from the night. Sink into a state of wonder. Marvel at the view.

creative dreamer

Dreams remind us that we each have an artist within us. After all, these creative productions come to even the most pragmatic person. So let your inner dream artist out: Draw your dream with colored pencils, or make a collage based on the themes, imagery, colors, or moods of your dreams. Write a dream poem, or sing and dance your dream's stories.

dream holiday

Special and momentous occasions, such as birthdays, the New Year, or the beginning of a new job or adventure, are all great times to ask your dreams for guidance. Write a question in your journal on the eve of any such event and invite your dreams to grace you with the gift of insight.

dreamy gifts

From time to time buy yourself a little present, such as a pendant, a piece of artwork, or an item of clothing based on a dream you've had. This gift to yourself can help remind you of the gifts of insight and understanding your dreams have delivered.

dream jokes

The dreaming mind is endlessly creative. Look for puns and plays on words in your dreams. The multiple meanings in a word may give you new ideas about what your dream wants to tell you.

• • • • • • • •

THE SOUND OF ONE MIND DREAMING

Think of your dream as a Zen koan: a kind of riddle or paradoxical teaching story given to meditation students to jolt them out of logical thinking and into epiphany, insight, or enlightenment. One well-known koan is, *What is the sound of one hand clapping?* The koan, like the dream, resists everyday linear thinking. It can be nonsensical or downright mystifying.

In this spirit, contemplate any dream with a spacious and open mind, allowing its wisdom to unfold on its own. Don't chase the meaning but instead let it sneak up on you. The answer will come when you've finally given up on expecting an answer. Then *voilà*! It appears as a splash of insight in a puddle of glitter and gold at your feet.

*Without leaps
of imagination,
or dreaming,
we lose the excitement
of possibilities.*

GLORIA STEINEM

YOUR BRAIN ON DREAMS

what science can — and can't — tell us

T his is an exciting time to study dreams and the unconscious. Brain imaging technology offers us new information about dreams, which In turn allows scientists and dream researchers to examine connections between brain activity associated with dreaming and the psychological and spiritual aspects of dreaming. Arising from this research are many compelling questions to ponder about our dreaming minds and our ever-evolving systems of belief regarding them.

Various scientific theories have been advanced to explain how dreams are formed. Among them is the idea that dreams are the result of neuronal firings that are then synthesized into image and story. This theory has been used by some to write dreams off as random hallucinatory narratives and justify a cultural shift away from exploring dreams as meaningful.

Interestingly, the dreaming brain is highly active, especially during the rapid eye movement (REM) sleep cycle. When we're awake, thoughts, attitudes, memories, and feelings result from brain activity; so, too, in REM sleep thoughts are being generated. However, in this case they bubble up from a different neurochemical stew, thus giving our mind, and the thoughts it produces, distinct characteristics as compared with the waking mind. If we see these alterations as imperfections, or evidence that the brain is simply firing on too few cylinders, it is easy to dismiss dream content and write it off. If, on the other hand, we accept dreaming as a different but still valuable form of consciousness, there is much to explore and discover.

Let's look at some of what brain science teaches us about our dreaming mind.

THE DREAMING BRAIN ISN'T SLEEPING. The brain is as active during REM sleep, the phase when most vivid dreams take place, as it is awake (and some brain regions are even more active when dreaming than when we're awake).

THE DREAMING BRAIN IS HIGHLY EMOTIONAL. Have you ever noticed that dreams are often intensely scary, exciting, or upsetting? One reason is that the limbic system, where our fight-or-flight reactions and strong emotions originate, is highly active when we're dreaming.

THE BRAIN DREAMS WITH ITS EYES OPEN. Even though our eyes are closed when we're asleep and dreaming, parts of the visual cortex are highly active during dreaming. No wonder dreams are filled with such rich and cinematic imagery.

THE DREAMING BRAIN HAS NO IDEA WHERE IT IS. The precuneus, the brain region that tells the body where it is located in space, is generally offline when dreaming, which is why you're usually not conscious of the fact that your body is at home in bed during your nocturnal adventures.

THE LOGIC BEHIND THOSE ILLOGICAL DREAMS. Ever wonder why dreams seem to operate in their own world of crazy logic? It's because at least two important regions that oversee continuity, short-term memory, and logic (the dorsal lateral prefrontal cortex, aka the DLPFC, and the precuneus) are deactivated while we dream. Thus, you might dream your college professor is dancing with your mother, even though the two of them never met in waking life.

THE DREAMING BRAIN DOESN'T KNOW WHERE IT LEFT THE CAR KEYS EITHER. Again, because the DLPFC and the precuneus are deactivated during REM sleep, we lack the ability to fully exercise our short-term memory when we dream. This might help explain breaks in continuity during dreams as well as why it's often difficult to recall dreams upon waking.

THE EXECUTIVE IS OUT TO LUNCH. Making decisions or directing our will is likewise difficult in most dreams. That's because the parts of our brain that control executive function are, well, asleep.

WHY DO WE DREAM?

While science can tell us what parts of the brain are active — or not — when we dream, science still can't say for certain *why* we dream. Nor can science define precisely what a dream is. (Nor what a thought is, nor what the mind is, for that matter.) But since everybody dreams, and an awful lot of brainpower is expended in the process, it seems logical to assume there are good reasons for why we dream away such a large portion of our lives. Here is some of what we *do* know about the effects of dreaming.

EMOTIONAL REGULATION. Dreams help us process the emotions of our daily lives.

PROBLEM SOLVING. Because the dreaming mind is adept at making random associations — bringing together surprising and seemingly unrelated people, events, and images — dreams help us solve problems and prepare us for insights and epiphanies.

REHEARSING FOR FUTURE EVENTS. Dreams allow us to try out possible strategies for situations we might face in waking life.

MEMORY CONSOLIDATION. Dreams are like a nightly janitor who disposes of unnecessary memories or an industrious librarian on the night shift who catalogs our memories, making room for new ones.

• • • • • • • •

IT'S ELEMENTARY

Science has come to be regarded as a rarefied branch of study exclusively for highly trained people, but, more broadly, science is just a way of being intentionally curious. After all, REM sleep was first discovered not using sophisticated lab equipment, but by simple observation. In 1953, scientists Eugene Aserinsky and Nathaniel Kleitman noticed the rolling movement behind the closed eyelids of sleeping infants, leading them to propose that dreams take place during what they called rapid eye movement sleep. They later used EEG monitors in the lab to confirm their theory.

Be your own sleep and dream scientist. Ask questions about dreams, get curious, take notes, and observe. The first step is to remember more dreams. This is a skill you can practice and improve on. Later in this section there will be suggestions on how to remember more dreams and more details from your dreams. For now, follow the instructions in this section to get started.

take notes

Journal about your dreams as well as about your waking experiences to begin to make observations and draw your own conclusions about dreams. Like a good scientist, date your entries, and make notes of any connections between your daytime activities and the themes and imagery that arise in your dreams. Review your journal monthly or quarterly, and take note of any intriguing insights or meaningful connections you make about your dreaming and waking experiences and how they impact one another.

attitude adjustment

Take an attitude of nonjudgmental curiosity and be open to what your dreams have to offer.

come in with questions

If you have a particular question about dreams, such as how what you eat affects your dreams, whether new ideas are sparked by your dreams, or even whether dreams come true in your waking life, track these questions in your journal, and make notations about what you observe.

• • • • • • • •

THIS I BELIEVE

Through years of personal experience, intensive study, and working with others and their dreams, I have come to my own beliefs about dreams:

GOOD GUYS. I believe that all dreams are good (yes, even nightmares). I have found that they contain useful information for us and that they always come to us in the service of health and healing.

DREAM DOCTORS. I believe dreams can aid in the diagnosis of illness and offer remedies for everything from cold and flu to chronic fatigue. My own dreams seem to specialize in nutrition: they accurately suggest foods I should eat more of and others I should avoid.

BFFS UNFILTERED. I believe dreams will tell it like it is — if only we'll listen. Like the best friend who will point out the spinach that's stuck between your teeth or a label peeking out from the back of your shirt, dreams don't let us fool ourselves into thinking we're doing better than we really are. And they're always there to help us become the very best version of ourselves. I have also found that dreams never criticize without offering constructive help in the form of images, puns, or stories that point us toward inner strengths and sources of sustenance and support.

INNER ORACLES. I believe dreams can help us access knowledge and wisdom that we are not aware of when awake. Dreams can offer guidance on everything from relationships to real estate. My own dreams have acted as personal coach, guru, matchmaker, and more.

CONNECTORS. I believe that dreams can bring us closer to our loved ones and the world. When I dream a friend or family member is in distress, I usually call them in the morning to see how they are doing. Nine times out of ten they tell me they really were going through something difficult and are so glad that I called. Through dreams I've also become more attuned to the moods and needs of my pets, and I have become more interested in the welfare of other animals, and even the environment.

When we are awake to our dreams, we also wake up our empathy, compassion, and curiosity, thus helping us feel more connected to others and to the world around us.

DREAM NOTATIONS

Now it's your turn. How have your dreams helped you? What do you believe their role is in your life? In the world? Write about it.

*The nicest thing for me
is sleep, then at least
I can dream.*

MARILYN MONROE

TRY TO REMEMBER

improving dream recall

In waking life we accept that we remember some things and forget others. But when it comes to dreams, we more or less expect to forget. Scientists tell us that low dream recall is the norm because the brain areas that support short-term memory are less active when we're dreaming. But there must be more to it than that. After all, in cultures that value dreams, people remember them on a regular basis and in detail — the way some of us can remember the batting averages of every Red Sox player that ever hit a ball, or lines from favorite songs we haven't danced to since the days of three-piece white suits and disco balls. But we live in a place and time when dreams are considered bizarre or random occurrences void of meaning, so perhaps it's not surprising that the general population tends not to remember them.

There are many factors that can interfere with dream recall, from medications or supplements to inadequate sleep and other physiological issues. However, simply by paying attention to our dreams, valuing them, and creating favorable conditions for sleep and dreaming, we can boost dream recall. By now we've touched on several reasons why it's worth the effort: Dreams give us fresh perspective, offer creative counsel, help us through tough times by offering insight, and even help ease or heal insomnia, especially for people who experience frequent nightmares and disturbing dreams. In addition, working with dreams in therapeutic settings has been shown to decrease anxiety and increase feelings of overall well-being.

But even if you have low dream recall, you can still reap many of the benefits that dreams offer. According to the Swiss psychiatrist Carl Jung — whose work defines much of our understanding of dreams — they help us integrate the information in our conscious and unconscious minds. Dreams help us evolve emotionally and spiritually, with or without dreamwork. That is, dreams are helping and supporting us in the background even if we don't remember them.

· · · · · · · ·

LOW RECALL? NO WORRIES

There is so much to remember every day: birthdays and anniversaries, passwords and PINs, not to mention where we left our keys and what we did with our eyeglasses — to name just a few. So it's no wonder that sometimes we can't seem to remember our dreams. If you have low recall, don't worry. Dreamwork techniques can still help you to grow and evolve in your life — and who knows, they may even help you find your glasses. Here are some ways to generate material you can use for dreamwork when you can't remember your dreams.

dreams have no expiration date

If you rarely record a dream and only remember a small handful from your life so far, continue to work on the ones you do remember using different techniques at different times. Chances are, you will continue to uncover more and more glints of psychological gold the more you work on a single dream, even one from the distant past.

pick a card

Purchase a deck of tarot cards that have vibrant, dreamy images, or create a file of unusual and compelling pictures clipped from magazines or brochures from art exhibits. Then, without looking, choose a card or picture that will serve as your dream. Trust the magic of chance to give you the "dream" you need in that moment. You can work with that image just as you would work with a dream (meditate on it, make associations to it, etc.), while receiving many of the same benefits from the process.

waking dreams work, too

Another option if you don't have a dream to work on is to choose an unusual or surprising event from your waking life to use as if it were a dream. For example, if a coyote ran in front of your car as you drove down the highway; your dishwasher, television, or something else you rely on broke; you had an accident or mishap; or you ordered a winter coat online but instead received a package that mistakenly contained a string bikini — any of these types of experiences could function as material to use for a dreamwork exercise.

*An uninterpreted
dream is like
an unread letter
from God.*

THE TALMUD

. . . .

HINTS FOR A HEALTHY DREAM HARVEST

Sometimes dreams behave like reticent teenagers. They withdraw and test us with their silence. But as every wise parent and caring teacher knows, if you stick with them and let them know you're listening, they'll start to share their wise, warm, and lovable selves with you. Patience helps with both teens and dreams. As for dreams, here are some tips to get them talking to you and to help you remember what they have to say.

build on success

Avoid making blanket statements such as "I don't remember my dreams." Not only will negative thoughts and statements negatively affect your dream recall, but also, such statements are likely untrue. Everyone dreams and nearly everyone remembers some dreams, even if they occurred in childhood. So start with what you do remember and build from there. You might even say, "In the past I didn't remember many dreams, but now I'm improving my dream recall." Give your subconscious a positive message about your intentions, and you'll be more likely to succeed in remembering.

take a genuine interest in your dreams

Read articles or books about dreams, ask other people about their dreams, and become curious about any dreams or dream snippets that you *do* recall, no matter how mundane they at first appear to be.

identify dream themes

Spend a moment in stillness before getting out of bed to allow any dream memories to come to you. If nothing comes to mind, give your memory a gentle nudge. Consider possible themes or characters you might have dreamed about based on relevant themes in your dreams or your waking experiences. For example, if you often dream of houses, water, or travel, ask yourself if any of these themes appeared in last night's dream. Or ask yourself if you dreamed of any people or situations in your daily life, such as work, family, or friends. Don't push for answers — simply invite possibilities, and see if something floats up to the surface.

keep the door open for dreams all day

If you don't remember a dream first thing in the morning, don't despair. Dream fragments, or even an entire scene, may come to you while you are doing something else entirely. The shower seems to be a good place for dreams to resurface, so be prepared! Your morning run, your commute to work, and other early activities are all times when dreams might pop back into your consciousness.

keep a dream journal

There's one nearly foolproof way to get dream recall flowing: at night, before bed, write down your intention to remember your dreams, and then record your dreams in the morning. Dreams can be hard to hold on to, so grab your journal first thing when you awake — even before you roll over and kiss your sweetie good morning — and write down whatever you remember. This simple routine tells your dreaming mind that you're serious about wanting to remember. Later I will offer more ways to make your dream journal a key part of your dreamwork (see page 99).

• • • • • • • •

THE KEY

At the end of a labyrinthine hallway, beyond courtyards, crypt-like spaces, and spiraling staircases, you find yourself at last before a great door looming large as a wall.

In your hand you hold a key: heavy, silver, and long enough to cross the entire palm of your hand. It looks like a child's stick-figure draw-ing of a person with a lollipop head on a long, narrow column of a body with a single flat, jagged foot splayed to one side.

On the door before you, two keyholes are stacked, one over the other, just above eye level. Not knowing which to choose, you jab the key uselessly at one and then the other, fighting the unseen inner cham-bers that refuse to roll themselves open into welcome. You try the key again and again, push then pull, then slide your bags from your shoulder and onto the cobblestone floor. Taking a deep breath, you try again.

The symbolism of doors that won't budge, and the jabbing and wrenching of skeleton keys that won't turn, is not lost on you, who have long immersed yourself in the alphabet of archetypes, image, and alchemy.

Finally, a robed figure appears out of nowhere, takes the key from your hand, glides it into the bottom lock, twists and pushes with unhurried force, and says simply, "Like this," before handing back the key and disappearing.

At last you can pass through the doorway marked Dreams. *You have come here to find meaning, guidance, and long-awaited answers. After frustrated effort followed by surrender, you see another door open into another chamber. At long last mastery seems possible.*

And then, three flights up, another locked door, another key in your hand . . . countless new challenges and a lifetime of dreams to unlock.

Yes, dear reader, we have arrived at that same door. Or, if not at a mystical magical door of dreams, we have arrived at least at this page, where you are hoping, I'm quite sure, that I'll hand you the key to unlocking the secret to dream interpretation.

If this is indeed what you are hoping, you are not alone. The phrase "dream interpretation" is typed into the Google search bar (our modern-day oracle, you could say) nearly 250,000 times a month. Indeed, there are a lot of curious dreamers out there.

What there *isn't*, however, is a fairytale brass key to unlock your dreams' meanings. Nor is there a plain silver house key or even an answer key. There is no one-size-fits-all interpretation for any dream, and you may as well put that dream dictionary away, too. Each dream is unique, and what meaning it holds depends on the dreamer's personal stock of memory, association, and countless experiences.

So rather than trying to reduce a dream to a single door needing to be opened with a specific key, or a puzzle to be solved, we'll regard each dream as a riddle whose purpose is to help us open up questions rather than close down discussions with simple yes or no answers.

When we stop jabbing impatiently at the dream and instead allow it to reveal itself in time, we can be dazzled by the ingenuity of the dreaming mind and receive its lessons with less effort. As in mindfulness meditation itself, we detach from the results of the practice, but commit to remaining aware, alert — and, yes, *awake* to the process itself.

some questions you might ask

To begin to unlock the myriad messages and meanings within your dreams, open up a dialogue with them. Here are some questions to get you started:

- What interests me most about this dream?

- What does this dream make me feel? Where do I experience that emotion in my body? Do I feel that way about anything in my waking life?

- What am I afraid of in this dream?

- What do I most want in this dream?

- Does this dream remind me of any situation I'm facing right now in my life?

- Mythologist Joseph Campbell has said that "Myths are public dreams; dreams are private myths." What is the underlying story or myth that your dream is telling?

*The interpretation of
dreams is the royal road
to a knowledge of the
unconscious activities
of the mind.*

SIGMUND FREUD

SLOW WAVE

taking time to understand your dream language

Dreamwork can take many forms, from talking about dreams to writing about them to creating art from them. And it need not be complicated. Simply taking the time each morning to recall and reflect on your dreams, whether or not you understand them, is the first step in creating a dreamwork practice that can sweeten your life. Sharing dreams with another person is also a form of dreamwork. More structured forms of dreamwork with therapists and analysts, either individually or in groups, are also available.

Taking a mindful approach to dreamwork means that we value the process of working with our dreams as much as the specific answers the dreams might provide. We give ourselves permission to spend relaxed and thoughtful time with our dreams, and we study them for the clues they give us about what is going on below the surface of our conscious thinking mind. Among other things, we notice the emotional tenor of the dream, its clarity or lack thereof, the beliefs that are exposed, and where the conflict lies within the dream. Each of these elements gives us information about the issues and emotions that need our attention in our waking life. We discover hints about emotional blocks, inner resistance, and outdated beliefs that may be holding us back from achieving our goals or stunting our emotional and spiritual growth.

As in mindfulness meditation, the act of turning toward dreams with curiosity and an attitude of openness helps us become self-aware and awake in daily life. As a result, we can reflect on — rather than react to — situations and events, and experience greater mental flexibility and more equanimity.

In the following pages I'll offer ideas and suggestions for you to experiment with so that you can learn to work effectively with your dreams. Try a few of these practices and see which work for you. Come back to this section from time to time and see if another idea, tip, or technique appeals to you; if so, try it out.

· · · · · · · ·

DREAMWORK WORKS

Dreamwork is a practical and effective way to get to know yourself more deeply and to achieve personal growth and healing. Therapeutic dreamwork has been shown to:

- Facilitate creative breakthroughs

- Aid in the grieving process

- Help people who are facing a life transition such as divorce, a career change, or a new stage of development

- Support physical and psychological healing

- Deepen intuition

- Heal nightmares

- And much more

· · · · · · · ·

SPEAKING OF DREAMS

Has anyone asked you about your dreams lately? If you're like most people these days, the answer is probably no. So, in addition to initiating an inner dialogue about your own dreams, as described above, initiate conversations with others about their dreams, too. Talking about dreams with loved ones has been shown to strengthen relationships. That may be because dreams come from deep inside, and they often reveal parts of ourselves we don't ordinarily show to others, and even aspects of ourselves that we haven't yet fully acknowledged. Discussing dreams helps us open up authentic lines of communication and therefore encourages closeness.

The key to healthy conversations about dreams — or anything else for that matter — is to listen with an open mind and a loving heart. When it comes to dreams, this is especially important. There is no need to analyze or interpret one another's dreams; being present is enough.

dream sharing

Ask a friend or family member how they slept and whether they dreamed. Don't pressure yourself to figure the dream out. Just bringing dreams out of the dark and into the daylight invites greater closeness and brings the dreams' creativity, humor, and surprising new perspectives into our lives.

kids' dreams count

Ask a child what they dreamed last night, and when they answer, listen with interest to what they have to say. Follow their lead about whether to pursue the discussion further. Simply by posing the question, you've opened the door to future sharing and shown that you value the inner life of imagination and emotion.

reach out

You need not wait for someone to inquire about your dreams. If you have an intriguing or important dream to share, call a friend or ask a family member to listen to you describe it. Better yet, find a dream group or identify a few people in your circle of contacts who share your interest in dreams, and agree to be there for one another when you have a dream you want to discuss.

*There is innately
in every human being
a desire to hear stories
that matter, and dreams
are stories that matter.*

CLARISSA PINKOLA ESTÉS

• • • • • • • • •

SAFETY IN SHARING

Sharing dreams requires a great deal of safety and trust. Here are some guidelines to follow when talking about dreams informally with friends and loved ones or in groups.

the vegas rule

What's said between dreamers stays with those dreamers. Observe strict confidentiality in all things dreamy.

the "aha!" moment

When talking about dreams, remember that there's not one right answer. Any answer that elicits an "Aha!" of recognition, the feeling that something has resonated inside, or a flash of insight is *one* of the right answers. Over time a single dream can reveal various facets and new bits of information and meaning may emerge.

no dream 'jacking

Don't hijack someone else's dream by telling them what it means or how they should interpret it. Instead, listen to the dream as if it were your own. Then use the phrase "If it were my dream" to introduce your comments about it. Remember, the only interpretation that matters is the one that resonates with the dreamer.

job description

When someone shares a dream with you, it's not your job to offer answers or solve puzzles. Your job is to listen and reflect back what you hear. Simply by tuning into the dream with open-minded curiosity, you help create the conditions for the dreamer to have their own insights about it. And that's what counts.

• • • • • • • •

SYMBOLICALLY SPEAKING

Sometimes I feel so perplexed by a dream that I find myself sputtering, "Why can't this dream just speak to me in plain English?" On days like that, I wish I had one of those decoder rings I used to dig out of the bottom of a cereal box or order from the back of a comic book. In this case, the little plastic trinket would translate my dream for me in one fell swoop. Of course there is no such handy-dandy dream decoder ring. But there are many ways to approach a dream that can coax the dream's messages to the surface. Here are a few to get you started.

let the dream speak

Random neuronal activation may have created the impulses that formed the basis of your dream, but the mind's synthesis of those impulses ensures that the dream is anything but random. In fact, Carl Jung maintained that every element of a dream is in place for a reason and has meaning.

The following exercise, inspired by Robert Hoss's "The 6 Magic Questions" in his book *Dream Language*, can help you unearth the information and wisdom encapsulated in each image in your dream. You can do this alone or with a partner.

Choose an inanimate object from your dream (this can be anything from a solid object such as a pitcher or table, to something less concrete such as the rain or wind). Then follow these steps:

1. Get still and quiet by taking a few long, slow breaths as you relax your body and mind. Then, bring your dream object to mind. Observe it closely, using all five senses. When you can see it clearly, imagine that you are this thing. Fully experience what this feels like.

2. Complete these statements (don't think too hard, just go with your first response) as if you are that object:

   I am a _____

   My purpose is _____

   What I like best is _____

   What I dislike most is _____

   What I fear most is _____

   What I desire most is _____

   I have come to tell you _____

3. When you have completed the questions, say goodbye to the dream object you've been embodying, and come back to yourself. Take a few breaths to settle into your body, once again feeling your feet on the floor, the air on your skin, and return to noticing the sounds around you.

4. When you are ready, read the statements in step 2 and consider these questions:

    Are any of these statements true for you? If yes, does the statement refer to an aspect of your life, a problem, or an issue you are facing?

    If the statement is positive, can you use it as an affirmation — a reminder of your strengths or positive attributes?

    If the statement is negative, can you view it from a new perspective to find a lesson or strength in it?

    What concrete action can you take to incorporate your new awareness into your life?

> *Be patient toward all
> that is unsolved in your heart
> and try to love
> the questions themselves.*
>
> RAINER MARIA RILKE

. . . .

PARTS OF MYSELF

Sometimes it seems like it would take a village to help you understand a single dream. Luckily you've got one — right inside your head. You might be familiar with the concept of the inner child: the 4-year-old who still lives inside your 50-something-year-old body and who is still upset, for example, that her mother wouldn't let her buy the blue polka-dot dress she wanted so badly. Long after you've outgrown your affection for polka dots, you can still feel the sting of that denial. Well, that's not all. In addition to that inner 4-year-old, you have an inner rebel and an inner saint, an inner recluse and an inner cocktail-party hostess. Okay, maybe not a cocktail-party hostess, but you get the idea.

If it seems strange to think about having a cast of characters living inside you, think of all the ways we acknowledge this on a regular basis. When we say, "Part of me wants to eat that ice cream sundae, but part of me wants to be able to fit into my bathing suit, so I'm going to say no," or when we can't make a decision and say, "I'm of two minds on that," we're working to assimilate different parts of our personality.

As long as we're able to negotiate with these various voices, there's no problem. But sometimes, rather than negotiate, we negate. We don't like that tantrum-throwing 2-year-old who starts clenching her fists and bawling when we need to work late, so we confine her to a corner of our unconscious and plow ahead with that 10-hour workday. But guess what? None of these parts go away. So that toddler you've tried to banish might just show up as a shady character chasing you down a dark alley in a dream one night. These repressed and rejected parts of ourselves are what Jung referred to as our "shadows." They show up in dreams as dirty, mean, scary, and repulsive dream characters.

Some of us even reject our better selves. Maybe we think we don't deserve to do well or that putting on beautiful clothes or makeup is just a sign of vanity, so we stick to a wardrobe designed to conceal our unique style rather than reveal it. In our dreams a glamorous movie star might show up to remind us of the shimmering appeal that is part of us, too. You might call this your golden shadow, the part you aspire to but haven't yet been able to fully express.

The goal of dreamwork is to bring the many parts of yourself into harmony and to let each one have its say. Ultimately we want to find healthy outlets and positive forms of expression for aspects of ourselves that we have shunned.

all together now

Dreamwork is a great way to get acquainted with the various characters that inhabit your subconscious — and to help them all get along with one another. Here's an exercise to get you started:

1. Choose one to three characters from a dream. They can be people you know in waking life or characters that exist only in the dream. Either way, write down the character's name (if you know it) or any identifying label (cook, teacher, or woman in blue dress, for example).

2. For each character list three personality traits or qualities that come to mind when you think of that person. Go with the first three things that come to mind. There are no wrong answers here.

3. Now, review those characteristics. Notice the ways you are like this dream character and how you are different.

4. Next, reread the dream as if this character is a part of you. If in the dream you were fighting with your best friend who is artistic, flighty, and generous, consider whether in your waking life you are struggling in some way with the part of yourself who is artistic, flighty, and/or

generous. Is there a way that you are in conflict with your own inner artist? Are you being stingy in some part of your life?

5. Use the information you gain from this exercise to take some action to bring yourself into balance. If the dream is showing you that you're in conflict with your inner artist, for example, maybe it's time to sign up for a watercolor class or take out your colored pencils and draw.

· · · · · · · · ·

THE SKELETAL DREAM

When it comes to dreamwork, sometimes less is more. In this exercise you will strip the dream of description, commentary, and emotion, paring it back to its essential storyline. In this way you can get in touch with the essence — or the bones — of the dream. You can do this alone or with a partner. Here's how:

1. Write down the bare bones version of your dream, stripped to its most basic elements. Include actions and generalized descriptions. Eliminate details, including emotions and any editorializing.

   For example, rather than say,

   > I am being chased down a deserted alley in a city that looks a little like New York. My pursuer is a burly man, scary looking, wielding a club of some sort . . .

   Pare it back to

   > I am being chased by something big and scary.

2. Read the stripped-down version of the dream aloud to yourself or your partner.

3. Now ask yourself how the skeletal version of your dream resonates with your waking life. For example, you might find that the dream of being chased by something big and scary reminds you of how you feel about an impending deadline or another life situation that you are emotionally or metaphorically "running away from."

4. Once you've identified what waking life situation the dream might be alluding to, create an action step you will take to integrate what you've learned from the dream. In the example above, you might talk to your boss about the difficulty you're having making your deadline, or simply change your attitude toward the deadline by reminding yourself of your strengths and any support you have that will help you meet it.

*A writer
manufactures
a dream.*

ANTHONY DOERR

ZEN AND THE ART OF KEEPING A DREAM JOURNAL

The dream was fixed in my mind even before I opened my eyes. In it, I was lost and searching for a Japanese restaurant called Zen, where I eat from time to time in waking life.

I woke that morning in a hotel in Charleston, South Carolina, where I was attending a seminar on dreams. I'd been remembering an average of six to eight dreams a night, plus recording them in my journal. My waking life was no less busy. I was working, studying for my dream certification, and helping to care for my aging mother. So on this particular morning, I was not only tired, but I was also tired of recording all those dreams. Besides, I'd overslept a bit, so I was already running late. I had emails to answer and phone calls to make before I was scheduled to have breakfast and meet up with my class. I considered skipping my morning dream-recording ritual just this once. But out of habit I opened my notebook, picked up my pen, and began to write: "I am lost and looking for Zen."

As I wrote those words I smiled in recognition. Yes, it was true! In the dream I was lost and looking for Zen, the Japanese restaurant, but more broadly, in my working life I was lost in busy-ness and to-do lists, appointments and projects.

The dream announced the news of my life at that time: I was lost and looking for Zen. I needed the feelings of clarity and inner spaciousness that I associate with that philosophy. I needed hours in which to stretch out on the sofa with a good book, reading and dozing — or just plain doing nothing.

If I hadn't written the dream out, I would have kept running on autopilot, and I would have missed the dream's message. At that rate I might have gotten sick or had an accident, which is how the body grabs our attention as a last resort when we haven't listened to the more subtle messages it has been sending, asking us to slow down.

That morning I recommitted to meditating for at least 12 minutes a day, and blocking out time each day for "doing nothing." But first, I picked up the remote control and decided to stay in bed a half hour longer to enjoy a little TV, even if that meant I'd be late for my first meeting. After all, the moment one knows they are lost, they are already on the road to being found.

• • • • • • • •

THE MAGIC (OF) WORDS

Why is it that writing is so often the magic ingredient that brings a dream from mystery to meaning? The concept makes no sense on first examination. The dream, after all, swims in a subterranean sea, a primal yet highly evolved world indifferent, for the most part, to written language.

With our eyes closed, asleep in our beds, we experience our dreaming mind feeling its way along the seabed of consciousness, reading the braille of our memories and emotions. In the morning we surface and, pen in hand, we lay the dream down word by word, as if lining up rows of shells harvested from the depths so they can glisten in the sun.

Writing the dream unifies us: Left Brain, meet Right Brain. Amphibious Mind, meet Rational Mind. The writing hand swirls these states of consciousness together into spiraling eddies, from which the wisdom of the dream emerges.

So pick up your pen, open your journal, and start writing. That riffling ocean of pages is calling you.

a minute for dreams

If you had dreams, but don't have time to write them out in full, list at least one dream headline for each. For example: "Chased by a Spider," "Faulty GPS," or "White Deer on Garden Path." If you don't remember any dreams, write down your impressions and memories about the night. Did you sleep restlessly or well? Did you get up? Did your cat snuggle up on the pillow with you? What did you experience?

on the other hand

One way to connect with the dreamy aspects of yourself — the unexpected bits of wisdom and insight that often come through in dreams — is to write with your nondominant hand. This is a highly simplified take on a complex topic, but the bottom line is that when you write with your nondominant hand (the left hand if you're a righty and vice versa), you are stimulating the other half of your brain, thus accessing new information and fresh perspectives. Also, writing your dreams this way will slow you down so you notice things you might otherwise have rushed past. You can also try writing down questions you have about the dream with your dominant hand, then answering them with your nondominant hand.

· · · · · · · ·

THE DREAM REPORT

Thanks to ever-improving technology, these days we can share images, video, or sound recordings of nearly anything we experience. But with all our gadgets and electronic wizardry, we still can't bring back so much as a snapshot of a dream. Writing it down lets us hold on to the ephemeral experience of our nightly adventures so we can remember and reflect on them. What follows are some basic guidelines for recording dreams in your journal.

what's the headline?

Just like giving a title to a poem or story, writing your dream headline helps you home in on the most important action or aspect of the dream. Giving your dream a headline or title also helps you quickly locate a dream when you are looking back in search of patterns or themes.

be present

Write your dream report in the present tense, as if it is happening right now. This will help you stay tuned in to the dream and continue to experience it and learn from it as you record it.

just the dream, please

In your dream report, focus on the dream itself, leaving any commentary or associations until later.

details, details

Write the dream in as much sensory detail as you can. Include the actions in the dream, the quality of light, the weather, the colors, the sounds, and so on. The more you practice noticing, the more you will notice.

feel it

Dreams speak primarily in image and emotion, but sometimes it is hard to identify exactly what the emotions are. Give yourself a few moments to reimagine yourself inside the dream, and consider which of the four primary emotions (glad, mad, sad, scared) comes closest to what you felt in the dream. Also record the emotion you felt upon waking from the dream.

end it

When you've finished writing down your dream report, mark the end with the initials EOD (for "End of Dream"). This will help separate the dream from any reflections or other writings that follow.

going beyond the basics

When a particular dream feels significant, or if you just want to explore more, reflect on the following aspects of your dream in your journal:

IMAGES. Each dream image contains within it your personal associations and memories, as well as a basic emotion. List up to five images from your dream and write a few words about what relevance each one has for you. What memories, thoughts, or feelings come up when you consider each one?

ASSOCIATIONS. Make note of any elements in your dream that remind you of situations in your waking life, from either the recent or distant past. Also consider whether you are likely to encounter some of these situations in the future. This can give you a hint about what part of your life the dream is referencing.

GUIDANCE. According to Jung, dreams come to us from the true Self, the core of our being, the part that guides us toward balance and wholeness. What direction is this dream, this message from the Self, pointing you in? Is it showing you a place where you are out of balance? Is it suggesting that you consider an aspect of yourself you've been neglecting or ignoring?

> *Finish this sentence: In order for me to be healthy, whole, and complete, my dream may be suggesting that I* _____.

ACTION. Although we sometimes use the word *dreamer* to describe someone who has his or her head in the clouds, active dreamers take guidance from their dreams and incorporate new insights into their daily lives. In this way, your personal evolution toward health and wholeness is empowered and enhanced by the dream. What small action can you take based on your dream?

> *Finish this sentence: I will honor my dream today by taking this small step:* _____.

MAKE IT POSITIVE. Create a positive statement or intention based on your dream. Make it short and direct like something you might read on a bumper sticker. Keeping it concise will help you remember it. You can also copy it onto an index card and post it where you will see it and be inspired by it.

• • • • • • • •

A PRACTICE TO PERFECT

Despite what the old saying promises, practice doesn't always make perfect. But devoted practice does increase the possibility of tapping into your greatest potential.

A practice is any habit that we commit to for the benefit of self-growth, emotional fulfillment, or spiritual fulfillment. Don't get hung up on trying to complete the journaling prompts perfectly. Instead, aim for perfect attendance (or close to it) by just showing up at the page. Think of this as a time to commune with, play with, learn from, and honor — both awake and dreaming.

*No one has known
himself truly
who has not studied
his dreams.*

SWAMI SIVANANDA

*In truth
it matters little
how far you can bend forward
or how far you can twist,
for wherever the point of
resistance lies is the place
where you have the greatest
opportunity to learn
and to change.*

DONNA FAHRI

THE YOGA
OF DREAMS

Not long after I began practicing yoga, and just as I was getting the hang of downward-facing dogs and sun salutations, I realized I was in trouble. While my alignment on the mat was quickly improving, I realized I might be out of alignment when it came to the spiritual teachings behind the practice.

To transcend the state of *maya* (illusion) and reach enlightenment, my yoga teachers explained, we must shake off the dream of this world. Further, our sleeping visions are merely dreams within a dream, which I understood to mean that they threatened to pull us even farther from the awake and aware state we were seeking. Then I learned that some yogic masters subsist on but a few hours of clear and dreamless sleep each night.

Here I was, an aspiring yogini who remembered several dreams each morning, who needed a good eight hours of sleep each night, and who looked to her dreams for guidance. The clarion call in the yoga community was, "Wake up! Wake up!" But rather than pull me away from my dreams, practicing yoga and meditation has helped me articulate and fine-tune my dreamwork practice. Dreams are, after all, a nightly invitation to a spiritual training ground that can be as rigorous and rewarding as a master yoga class.

Sure, one day perhaps I'll reach enlightenment and my mind will settle into dreamless clarity, both awake and asleep. But until then, I dwell in the understanding that paradoxically — and profoundly — the dreams we encounter asleep can provide the insight we need to move toward the ultimate goal of waking up into enlightenment.

• • • • • • • •

SOFTEN YOUR RESISTANCE — ON THE MAT AND ON THE PILLOW

In yoga class the teacher invites you to bend your body into seemingly impossible contortions. Then, when your muscles burn and you are about to give up, she offers instructions like, "Notice your body's resistance, bring your breath to that area, and on the exhale, soften and release." Her voice is soothing and consoling, but you can't imagine how any of this will help calm your quivering muscles or convert this uncomfortable pose into something that resembles grace or ease. Meanwhile, all you want is to sink into savasana, but what choice do you have? So you go ahead and do what the teacher says, and after several more classes you can touch your toes, arch into a backbend, or sit in full lotus position.

Just as a challenging yoga pose can show us where our muscles are tight or our bodies are out of alignment, so too can our dreams show us where we are resisting or in conflict with our soul's purpose or our heart's mission. If we are awake to our dreams, we can use what they bring forth from our subconscious to soften and release outdated beliefs about ourselves and the world.

For example, when in the dream world you find yourself face to face with a monster, an enemy, or a character you have nothing but scorn for, rather than flee, wake yourself up, or dismiss the dream as too disturbing to bother with, try turning toward the difficulty instead. Follow the same instruction that helped you find ease on the yoga mat and stay with the discomfort. Soften and release.

By working with your dreams using the techniques offered in this book, you will discover the healing messages in your dreams and improve your mental flexibility and emotional balance.

stretch with your dreams

Find a quiet place to settle in with your dream journal for 20 minutes or half an hour. Choose a dream to study and look for the point of resistance or conflict in it. Now, settle into a calm, centered mental attitude by taking some deep, slow breaths. When you are ready, pick up your journal and pen and begin an imaginative dialogue with your dream antagonist. Find out what he or she really wants from you. What can this dream character teach you?

Yes, answering this question can be even harder than enduring the burn of a difficult yoga pose. Just remember what the yoga teacher says, and breathe into the discomfort, soften and release your resistance. In time, practicing this type of dreamwork will help you become increasingly flexible — emotionally, mentally, and spiritually.

core muscles

In yoga, we do exercises to build our core muscle strength. In dreamwork, we exercise our emotional and spiritual muscles by engaging with the conflicts that arise in our dreams. By staying with the difficult scenarios presented to us, and considering all points of view offered up by the dream, we soften our identification with ego and start to align with our center, or core beliefs. This is an evolved stance, which is expansive, nonjudgmental, curious, and joyful.

take a breath

Breathing easily during sleep can help reduce the incidence of nightmares and soften their impact. Clear breathing also supports clear dreaming. The classic posture of sleeping on your side, with legs drawn up into a relaxed fetal position, hands in prayer position beneath or beside your ear, is a good option for creating a long spine and healthy breathing through the night.

dreaming hands

You can adapt *mudras*, or symbolic hand gestures practiced in yoga and meditation, to support your intentions to sleep and dream well. *Anjali* mudra, in which the hands come together in prayer position, is a common one for sleep. Placing our hands consciously into this position can help tap into the healing properties of the mudra, which is practiced to connect with the divine spark within. It is also seen as a gesture of harmony, bringing the left and right sides of the body together. To use this hand position to bring more intention and ease to your sleep and dreams, try this:

1. Lie on your back in bed and place your palms together in front of your heart, with fingertips gently touching. Maintain a little space between your palms, just big enough to hold a small imaginary flower blossom or feather.

2. With the sides of your thumbs resting against the center of your chest, breathe into your heart with several long, slow breaths, and feel the connection between your hands and your heart, your heart and your source.

3. Set an intention for your dreams. You might ask for soothing dreams, dreams of love, or guidance on a specific topic.

4. Now roll over onto your side, with hands remaining in *anjali* mudra. Find a comfortable spot for your hands, directly beneath your cheek, beneath your pillow, or slightly out in front of you on the mattress between your head and heart.

5. Focusing on your intention, allow yourself to drift into sleep and dreams.

the spirit of savasana

At the end of yoga class, we lie down in savasana pose to allow the benefits from the postures we practiced to settle into the body. Similarly, at the onset of sleep we can lie on our back or side, relax our muscles completely, and let go of our day. In this posture — both physical and mental — we stop worrying and pondering and instead trust the body, mind, and spirit to bring our deepest wisdom to bear on any unsolved issues or problems from the day. We trust they will be handled by our subconscious mind without any more conscious effort on our part.

with one eye open

According to various spiritual traditions, the spot on the forehead where the eyebrows meet, often referred to as the "third eye," is said to be the energetic center for inner vision and true insight. Once you are in bed with your eyes closed, relax the skin on your forehead and your eyelids, soften your eyes, and rest your attention gently on this third eye. Invite true insight to open within you, as you close your physical eyes to sleep and dream.

*The strangest things
are there for me,
Both things to eat
and things to see,
And many frightening
sights abroad
Till morning in the
land of Nod.*

ROBERT LOUIS STEVENSON,
FROM "THE LAND OF NOD"

NAVIGATING NIGHTMARES

when bad dreams happen to good people

You couldn't pay me to go into one of those haunted houses where zombies dripping with fake blood throw rubber snakes and spiders at visitors. And forget scary movies. I avoided watching *The Godfather* for decades all because of that one famous scene with the horse's head. I can't even watch the news after sunset. In short: I don't do scary.

But as someone with very high dream recall, I don't really get a choice when I close my eyes and go to sleep. Every night it's as though I'm entering a multiplex — only I didn't get to pick which movie I'm going to see. One night I might dream Antonio Banderas is sweeping me off my feet, and the next night I've got a starring role in *A Nightmare on Elm Street*.

I know I'm not alone in this. Between 5 and 6 percent of all dreams are nightmares, and, according to the American Sleep Association, up to 90 percent of us will experience a nightmare at least once, and most of us will experience them more often than that. But knowing that you're in good company when it comes to nightmares doesn't make them any easier to deal with. People often say they'd prefer not to remember their dreams at all, rather than risk remembering an occasional nightmare.

It's important to remember that when I say all dreams come to us for health and healing, I mean *all* dreams. Even nightmares. Especially nightmares. Not only that, working with nightmares can teach us how to live our lives with greater courage and grace. Dreamwork teaches us that so-called bad dreams are urgently trying to get our attention to help us face something we've been avoiding. When we learn to turn toward these scary dreams rather than ignore them, we can access their wisdom. This same process can also help us face scary situations when we're awake.

For example, when doing dreamwork on a scary dream, we might invent superpowers to help us face tidal waves, battles, or freefalls. Awake, too, we can identify superpowers, or special strengths that can help us confront looming problems. Okay, you may not be able to take down an attacker twice your size like you did in your dream or in the active imagination exercise you did during a dreamwork session, but maybe the process reminds you that you are stronger in spirit and heart than you thought you were. Admittedly you can't leap over tall buildings in a single bound when awake, but maybe your dream prompts you to call on the power of resiliency. In the dream you might fly away from danger, but awake you can defy the gravity of a situation by lightening up or taking a creative approach.

Working with your nightmares can teach you not to close your eyes to problems, sleepwalk through uncomfortable relationship issues, or be passive in the face of an unfulfilling job. Taking a lesson from nightmares and facing not only the frightening dream but also the uncomfortable thought or the thorny situation when awake can help you be a more active cocreator of your best dreams and your best waking life.

Yes, sometimes your dreams will lay it out on the table with painful urgency — but you can trust that there's loving intent behind the disturbing imagery with which the message may be delivered. Yup, even that nightmare that shook you awake.

That's why I encourage you not to just splash some cold water on your face, reassure yourself it was "only a dream," and go back to sleep. Dismissing these dreams altogether is a lost opportunity, because unlike cheesy horror movies, nightmares are actually inviting you to wake up to important truths about your life. If you can muster the courage to pay attention to them, discuss them with a friend or therapist, or do some dreamwork with them on your own, you will likely find the gift in the nightmare that makes the heart-stopping fear that woke you in the wee hours worth the price of admission.

SERIOUSLY BAD DREAMS

Luckily, for most adults, nightmares are infrequent episodes that don't interfere with getting a good night's rest. But for a small percentage of the population, nightmares are chronic and require professional attention. If you experience nightmares on a regular basis, and if they are affecting your ability to sleep or to function during the day, consult a doctor or therapist. In addition to medical treatments, there are proven methods for healing nightmares through dreamwork and different psychotherapeutic approaches — such as imagery rehearsal therapy — and other techniques.

SET THE SCENE FOR SAFE DREAMING

While most of the time our dreams will be benign — or even blissful — from time to time, we will all encounter one that wakes us up, heart racing, breathless, to reach for the light (both literally and figuratively). If nightmares or fear of the dark make bedtime scary for you, consider these tips for creating a sense of safety and protection at night.

protect the portals

Before bed, as you check to make sure the doors are locked and the shades and curtains are drawn, you can consciously create a cozy and safe environment for sleeping by affirming that you are symbolically closing the door on worries beyond your immediate control and sealing in your desire for inner peace. While you're no longer a child who's afraid of things that go thump in the night, this nightly routine, done with intention, is a signal to your subconscious that you're preparing a quiet, protected space for sleep and dreams.

comfort close at hand

Who says teddy bears and lullabies are just for kids? With or without plush toys, you can create an environment that feels safe and snuggly. This can help comfort you if you wake from a bad dream. Keep a picture nearby of a person or a place that makes you feel safe, or keep an extra pillow or two to cuddle up with when you wake up scared.

say your prayers

You don't have to be religious to express gratitude for the blessings in your life and ask for protection and guidance as you enter the realm of dreams. Say a prayer that aligns with your beliefs. Or, as you drift to sleep, simply affirm that you'll be safe and protected, and that your dreams will come in the service of love, goodness, and healing.

• • • • • • • •

MAKING THE MOST OF UNINVITED DREAM GUESTS

Let's face it, no one exactly rolls out the welcome mat and invites bad dreams in. But when they do come, don't slam the door shut and hope they'll skulk off for good, either. Taking just a little time to work with nightmares can do a world of good. Here are a few ideas for approaching nightmares and turning them from adversaries to allies.

have faith

When you wake from a nightmare, try to remember that all dreams work in the service of health and healing. While you're waiting for your heart rate to return to normal, reassure yourself that by light of day you might just find the healing message in the scary dream that shook you awake.

use your imagination

If during a nightmare you become lucid enough to think, "This is a dream, I am going to wake myself up," instead use your dreamy imagination to conjure up whatever you need to be safe and strong in the dream environment. For example, call on an animal helper, a superpower, a suit of armor, or whatever you need to emerge victorious. Then, turn and face the scary beast, pursuers, or enemy in your dream. Most likely that will be enough to send your fears scrambling for cover and leave you safe to dream brighter dreams.

call on the power of love

The best superpower in the dream world is the power of love, good, or God. Announce to your dream adversary that you are armed with one of these. You may neutralize your foe — or even turn him or her into an ally.

hit replay

If you are unable to take the types of actions suggested above when you are dreaming, try them when you're awake. Create a safe environment in which you have a dialogue with the scary elements in the dream, so you can find out what they want from you or what they have come to tell you. Imaginatively call in whatever helper, weapon, or scene change you need so you can face the dream again. Replay the dream by slowly writing it out in your journal or by calling it to mind and re-viewing it during meditation. Then, when you get to the scary part, alter the dream so that it resolves in your favor — or, if possible, for the good of all involved. You will know you have hit on an effective resolution when you feel calm and at peace in your body.

SCARY STORIES

Some of our favorite creepy tales (*Frankenstein*, *The Strange Case of Dr. Jekyll and Mr. Hyde*, and *Twilight*, to name a few) are really just recycled nightmares.

Try this: Take one of your scary dreams and write it out as if it were a story. One easy way to get started is to give any dream characters that you know from waking life (including yourself) new names, and instead of writing in the first person (using pronouns like "I" and "we"), write in the third person (using pronouns like "he," "she," "it," and "they"). Casting the nightmare as a story helps put some distance between yourself and the dream, which can help you gain insight into it. Plus, who knows, you may even get a best-selling book or screenplay from it!

· · · · · · · · ·

THE DARK SIDE OF DREAMS

Dreams famously bring to the surface thoughts and feelings we've repressed or rejected during the day. So it's not surprising that confrontations, various forms of violence, and even death are common themes. When they crop up in your dreams, consider the following ideas to help you make sense of them and uncover helpful messages — even in the most frightening dream.

what if i dream someone dies?

Dreams are rarely literal; more often they speak in metaphor. Thus, death in a dream may symbolize the death of an unhealthy attitude or a way of thinking or behaving that no longer serves you. It could even represent the end of a relationship or of some aspect of a relationship. Nightmares of widespread death or destruction could indicate the end of a worldview you've been holding on to that has ceased to be helpful.

If you dream that someone is trying to kill you or that someone is dying or being killed, ask yourself what part of yourself is ready to "die" or be released. However, if you sense that the dream is literally warning you about something, by all means check it out! Dreams work on many levels, and it's wise to consider all possible meanings.

night fights

Look at violent conflicts in your dreams as conflicts between parts of yourself that might be waging a metaphoric war within you. Are you fighting against a life situation? Are competing desires waging a war within you? What would each party need in order to accept a truce? Can you imagine a creative scenario in which these warring factions make peace? What action can you take in waking life to support this move toward equanimity?

If you dream you are being chased, ask what is pursuing you in waking life. You could be anxious over a deadline, or maybe there's an emotion you've been suppressing, a relationship issue you are neglecting to confront, or an area in your life you are not tending to. Rather than run away, ask yourself, "What would I learn if I faced this head on?" Remember, all dreams can help you find balance and wholeness in your life.

*In forming a bridge
between body and mind,
dreams may be used
as a springboard
from which man can leap
to new realms of experience lying
outside his normal state
of consciousness.*

ANN FARADAY

THE PLACES YOU'LL GO

taking dreaming
to the outer limits

You realize you can levitate and float to the ceiling. You sprout wings and become an iridescent blue butterfly. You are greeted by the captain of a spaceship who takes you on a journey to distant moons.

All of these experiences have happened in dreams. However, people tragically risk their health, well-being, and reputation to experiment with mind-altering substances just to have similar psychedelic escapades. We are drawn to transcendent experiences because we suspect there is more to life than what our senses can perceive, and we want to go beyond the boundaries of day-to-day existence to discover what else is possible. But it's not necessary or advisable to use dangerous substances to fulfill this desire. Happily, dreams can get us where we want to go safely.

Transcendent dreams can nurture our belief that we live in a conscious and responsive universe. They can make our lives feel richer, more magical, and more meaningful. Having extraordinary dreams, and welcoming their lessons, puts us in touch with a world of imagination and possibility that invites us to think deeper, live bolder, and dream bigger. Engaging with these extraordinary dreams can also increase our sense of presence, curiosity, wonder, and joy.

. . . .

ABSOLUTELY ORDINARY EXTRAORDINARY DREAMS

We say to our loved ones, "May your dreams come true," but when people report stories of times when they believe this has actually happened (for example that the events of a nighttime dream came to pass during the day) we often greet such stories with skepticism or outright disbelief. When pressed, however, even skeptics sometimes admit that they, too, have had a dream that defied logic or rational explanations. It might have been a dream of a deceased loved one that felt like a real encounter, or a dream that offered information they couldn't have consciously known about, or a dream that foretold a life event.

These types of dreams are not the exclusive domain of psychics or mystics. Everyday people often report having these remarkable dream experiences. Here are some of the types of extraordinary dreams that ordinary people encounter. Look through the list and make note of any you've experienced.

FALSE AWAKENING. You dream that you wake up in your normal surroundings, but then you realize that this too is a dream. This can be a disconcerting experience, but there is no cause for alarm. Soon enough you will wake in your real bed!

LUCID DREAMING. When you are aware within the dream that you are dreaming, this is called a lucid dream. This is a powerful dream state in which you can choose to direct your actions within the dreamscape.

DREAMS OF THE DECEASED. Dreams where we encounter a loved one who has died can be comforting, enlightening, or sometimes disturbing. Most of the time, however, the dreamer feels she has received a true gift of connection.

PRECOGNITIVE DREAMS. While many dreams incorporate people, places, and events from the past, the dreaming mind is in fact often looking to the future and playing out possible outcomes for the scenarios in our lives. When one of these comes to pass in waking life, we call it a precognitive dream.

BIG DREAMS. These are dreams that are memorable, and may stay with you for years, decades, even an entire lifetime. Big dreams often contain elements that go beyond your ordinary experiences and may take place in a different time period or unknown landscape. They may feature an archetypal figure like a priestess or sage and shimmer with a quality of luminescence or unusual clarity. Often they contain a message not only for you, the dreamer, but also for your family or the wider community.

SHARED DREAMS. On occasion, you might find that your dream is so similar to that of your bed partner or a friend that you have the feeling that you both visited the same location or shared an experience in the dream world.

MIX AND MATCH. Some dreams combine more than one category or are extraordinary for different reasons.

In your journal describe any extraordinary dream experience you've had.

*When one is asleep,
there is something in
consciousness which
declares that what
then presents itself
is but a dream.*

ARISTOTLE,
ON DREAMS

LUCID IS THE NEW BLACK

Not since the publication of Freud's *Interpretation of Dreams* in 1900, have so many people taken an interest in what goes on behind closed eyes. Lucid dreaming has made its way into movies, gone viral on YouTube, and become a social media darling. Indeed there are apps and gadgets that promise to jettison you into vivid lucid dreams whenever you want them.

It sounds crazy at first: With lucid dreaming, you know that you're dreaming, so rather than just being swept up in the action of the dream, you can make choices and do what you want. For instance, you can stand in your third-floor office and decide to fly out the window and take a tour of the treetops. You can hop a train in Duluth and travel directly to the Alps, or you can rub elbows with your favorite nineteenth-century poet.

Put simply, lucid dreaming is a hybrid state of consciousness in which you can simultaneously enjoy the creative brain chemistry of dreaming *and* facets of your daytime brain chemistry that allow you to make decisions, employ logic, and, importantly, know where your body is (asleep in bed), even while you remain in the dream doing all kinds of wild and wondrous things. Thus, you straddle two worlds.

If you've ever jolted yourself out of a scary dream because you suddenly realized, "This is a nightmare; I can wake myself up!" you've enjoyed a moment of dream lucidity. For just that instant before waking, you knew you were dreaming while you were dreaming. To fully experience lucid dreaming, however, rather than wake up, practice remaining in the dream while being conscious that you are dreaming.

If you've ever had one, you probably know why lucid dreaming is attracting so much attention. The awareness of having achieved lucidity is often accompanied by a wave of excitement, and you sense immediately that this is a precious state and it won't last long. To remain there requires the focus of a tightrope walker, so you slide your foot along the floor of the dream as every cell in your skin buzzes with the thrill. You feel more awake and alive than you ever have before — even while you're dreaming.

While many people induce lucidity to enjoy a playground of possibilities (flying, fabulous sex, tantalizing travel), the lucid dream state is also a powerful and creative state of consciousness that allows you to tap into healing powers, seek out information, solve problems, or see deeply into a situation you've been struggling with. A lucid dream is also like a laboratory where you can explore the dream state itself. You can interview dream characters and test the dreamscape to see what the wall, mountains, or waters are made of. You can even direct questions to the dream maker itself (your psyche, God, or simply the creative energy behind the dream, depending on your beliefs about where dreams come from).

directions to the land of lucid

Sometimes lucid dreaming "just happens," without any conscious effort on your part. But you can also learn to dream lucidly and to stay in the lucid state long enough to explore, play, heal, study, and learn.

WAKE UP. It's easier to have a lucid dream in the early morning hours, when REM periods (during which our most of our vivid dreams take place) are longer. To take advantage of this, drink a glass of water before bed to increase your chances of waking early, or set an alarm to rouse you an hour or two before you need to get up. When you wake, reaffirm your intention to have a lucid dream. Repeat to yourself, "I will become aware within my dream and know that I'm dreaming." This technique will increase your chance of having a lucid dream when you fall back to sleep — but you might want to try it only on nights when you can afford some disruption to your sleep.

BREATHE INTO IT. You can improve your chances of lucid dreaming by practicing gentle breath retention as you fall asleep or as you fall back to sleep after waking in the early morning hours (as described above). Prop yourself up on your pillows so you're sitting up in bed at a slight angle and try this:

1. Inhale slowly in for the count of four.

2. Gently retain your breath for the count of four.

3. Exhale slowly for the count of four.

4. Gently retain your breath for the count of four.

5. Continue this breathing pattern for several cycles as you ease into sleep.

go for the good

As with all experiences awake or asleep, go into lucid dreaming with an intention. Decide before bed what your goal will be once you achieve lucidity. We do our best soulful growth and healing in dreams if we affirm that we are using our dream explorations for the greater good, for love, and for healing. So always call on those powers when you make a request of the dream, and invite dreams that serve your highest and best good, as well as the highest and best good for all.

good
morning

. . .

I cannot be awake
for nothing looks to me as it did before,
Or else I am awake for the first time,
and all before has been a mean sleep.

WALT WHITMAN

It seems like it should be as simple as blinking your eyes open and feeling as bright as the morning sun. But it's all too common when the alarm rings to feel like you're prying your reluctant eyes open after a night that felt discouragingly short on sleep.

While the exercises and information about sleep and dreams in this book will help you wake with increased ease and alacrity, it's also important to note that what is going on behind your closed eyelids is no simple open and shut — or should I say shut and then open — routine.

›

Like a cat that has been left outside all night and is now pawing at the door to come in, you too must push through some resistance in order to enter the new day. In this case you must navigate cottony layers of dreams — not to mention some complex neurochemistry — to make your way back from the deep interiority of sleep to your familiar daytime surroundings of ticking clocks, tasks, and deadlines. In short, the parts of your brain that allow you to calculate, plan, and tend to logic and order are getting back to work — so that you can, too.

The body, also, must be coaxed back to life. Perhaps your sore neck or a stiff shoulder protests as you pull yourself up from prone to sitting. No wonder: your dreaming brain programmed you to forget your body for hours so you could be still and sleep safely. But now it's time to re-member yourself, wake up limb by limb.

In this section, we'll focus on taking a mindful approach to waking up, both in the simplest sense of getting out of bed — as well as in the deeper sense of tapping into present-moment awareness. That way you can step fully into each day, rather than risk sleepwalking through vast stretches of your life.

WIDE AWAKE

Notice what it's like for you to wake up in the morning. What thoughts fill your head? Worries? Wonder? What would you like to experience differently? Use these prompts to reflect on how you experience the morning.

> *When I wake up I tend to feel* _____.

> *If I could change one thing about the way I wake up in the morning it would be* _____.

> *If I woke up feeling more rested and refreshed, perhaps I could* _____
_____.

THE SILVER BALL

In most dreams, we're like the pinball in an arcade game, bouncing from thought to thought and from one mindless action to the next. We seem to be on autopilot with no way to direct ourselves and might experience it something like this:

> *Wow! I'm at school, and I'm in my pajamas. And now . . . suddenly I'm in a train station. I've got a knife in my hand. Now it's a plunger hoisted on my shoulder. I'm falling. I'm flying.*

Dreams can feel random and disjointed. This tumult of dream imagery might seem absurd, or even funny — except that if we aren't careful, our waking lives can feel equally disjointed. There may be days, or even weeks or months, during which we feel like we have surrendered our ability to direct our will and are again like that silver ball being flung around in some random pinball game. Our unchecked, reactive thoughts might flow something like this:

Someone's angry with me? Suddenly I'm angry now, too. The music on the radio swells, so now I feel uplifted. The corn chips are in a bowl on the table — I'm not hungry, but I'll eat a few handfuls anyway.

Just because our eyes are open and we've gotten out of bed doesn't mean we're necessarily awake in the true sense of the word. Paradoxically, we can learn a lot about waking up and living consciously and with intention by studying our dreams. As described earlier (page 127), when we wake up into a lucid dream, we realize that we have the power to make changes within the dreamscape. With this level of awareness, we can make choices instead of moving mindlessly through the dream.

We can take this lesson into our lives when we're awake, too. When we live lucidly, we can reflect rather than react. If someone hurts your feelings, you can choose to shake off the insult, rather than wear it around you like a heavy wool scarf on a summer day. If someone hits your car while you're stopped at a light, you can choose to boil over in anger or instead take a deep breath, assess what happened, and choose a reaction that will make the situation better, not worse.

What's more, when we become lucid within a dream, we often experience a rush of joy and even bliss as we recognize the unique state of consciousness we've achieved. In this way, lucidity shakes us into recognition of the precious nature of the dream state, thus heightening our appreciation of it. Waking up in the morning we also have the opportunity to become newly awakened to the precious nature of being alive.

As wide-awake dreamers, we cease being merely pinballed through life. Now we have our finger on the button. We can decide to merely flick that little silver ball of our volition or give it all we've got and try to light up the board. Or we can choose to keep the ball quietly and serenely in play.

. . . .

WAKE TO WONDER

You don't have to master the skill of lucid dreaming to bring more clarity and awareness to your experiences when awake. All you have to do is shift into present-moment awareness to become more clear and conscious — and fulfilled — all day long.

surprise!

It's the unusual things — the kitten that speaks, the bicycle that floats above the pavement, the familiar house that suddenly contains extra rooms — that alert us to the fact that we're in the rarified atmosphere of a dream. We can likewise use the appearance of seemingly illogical, unusual, or surprising events in our lives to wake us up to the wonder of any moment. Today, each time something out of the ordinary occurs, pause and shift your perspective slightly so you continue to see the ordinary but with extraordinary clarity and delight. That coin in your pocket, the watch on your wrist, the keys in your hand — let them all suddenly seem quite spectacular. Allow yourself to be surprised and amazed by the things you take for granted every day.

make it a mantra

"This is a dream!" we exclaim when we become lucid and aware within a dream. At that moment of recognition, the dream will often take on a quality

O wonder!
How many goodly
creatures are there here!
How beauteous mankind is!
O brave new world.

MIRANDA IN *THE TEMPEST*,
BY WILLIAM SHAKESPEARE

of ultra-real vitality and vibrancy. To remind yourself of the beauty of being alive, try using this related phrase as a mantra: "This is my life," or simply, "I'm alive!" Let these words remind you to look with fresh eyes at everyday marvels, such as the pattern and design that naturally appear in the wood grain of your kitchen table or floor, the branching veins within a single leaf, or the cascade of light and sound that's released when you turn on a faucet and water rushes down toward the drain. Suddenly an uneventful moment might just become a technicolor wonder.

am i awake or dreaming?

People who practice lucid dreaming ask themselves this question many times each day. The purpose is to help them remember, while they're awake, to ask the same question while dreaming in order to spark dream lucidity. But the same question can be asked by anyone at any time. Check in with yourself occasionally throughout the day, and ask yourself if you are awake and aware to the emotions and thoughts within you or if are you dreaming away the day by running on autopilot and missing out on the depths and details of your experience.

* * * * * * * *

YOU'VE GOT THE POWER

In this wide-awake dream we call life, too often we proceed like sleepwalkers, unconscious of our ability to call on our inner strengths and resources to influence the feeling-tone of our experiences. Yes, there is much that is beyond our control, but we all have the power to set intentions, to reflect before we react, and, best of all, to appreciate the dreamy world we have woken up to in our daily lives. Here are some ways you can use the wisdom of dreams to empower your life.

get active

Is there an area in your life where you can become a more engaged participant? Take a small step to make a difficult situation a little bit better, whether it's by shifting your attitude, finding the gift in the grief, getting support, or choosing love over fear when you make your next decision.

awake and aware

Be the witness today. Choose a situation to approach with the same engaged, nonjudgmental, open attitude that you use on the meditation cushion or in dreamwork. See what you learn when you listen with love and observe with empathy. Simply be present. No further action is required.

at the threshold

Just as it's advisable to set intentions for sleep and dreams before bed, it is just as important to set an intention before you enter each new day. Pause at the door of your bedroom and then again at the front door when you step outside. Each time, set or renew your positive intentions. Let each doorway remind you to check in with your desire to be awake and aware today. Pause, take a conscious breath, and proceed mindfully.

sync up with your dreams

One way to bring the magic of dreams into your day is to be alert to synchronicities. A synchronicity is defined as a remarkable confluence of events. A common synchronicity you have likely experienced is when you think of a friend you haven't seen or heard from in years and within hours she sends you a message or gives you a call. Or you dream about a hawk, and then, later, as you drive along the highway one swoops down in front of your windshield.

When we get in the habit of noticing synchronicities, our lives can take on a richer quality of flow and ease. Today, look for synchronicities, including echoes from dreams that show up in waking life. Take note of these in your journal and reflect on any meaning they might hold for you.

honor thy dream

When you remember a dream, honor it during the day by letting it inspire an action. For example, if the color red played a significant role in your dream, choose to wear a red shirt, scarf, or socks, and notice how that color makes you feel. If you dreamed of a cat that reminds you to connect with your intuitive side, stop and pet any cat you might encounter that day. If avocados appeared in your dream, have one in your salad at lunch, or research their health benefits. Find a fun, creative, safe, or even sacred way to bring a little piece of your dream into your waking experience. By honoring the dream in some small way, you keep the dream's wisdom close — and hasten its integration into your consciousness.

BED HEAD

waking the brain

In your dream, perhaps you were younger than you really are, or you were riding horses, which in waking life you never do. You might have been conversing with llamas or shaking out your golden locks (though your hair is midnight black). Then you wake up and settle back into your accustomed sense of your self, the one who matches (more or less) the picture on your driver's license.

Chronology snaps back to coherence with morning's light, and the logic of sequencing and continuity returns. While this all seems to happen in that first blink of your eyes, in fact behind the scenes a complex orchestration involving a dozen or more neurotransmitters and hormones is making it all possible. Serotonin and dopamine, acetylcholine, and norepinephrine are all coming back online as your brain shifts back to beta-wave thinking so you can reengage your wide-awake mind.

• • • • • • • •

THE SUN ALSO RISES

Just as the planets turn and the sun shines again each morning without any help from us, so too we shift from sleep and dreams to waking, whether we pay attention to the fact or not. But when we do so consciously, we have the opportunity to work with and enjoy the natural shifts in brain chemistry that wake us up each day. Here are some ideas to help you make the most of each new dawn.

there's a word for that

Dorveille is the French word for the liminal space between sleep and waking. Scientists call it "the hypnopompic state." Either way, this is a time when your mind is moving from the creative neurochemical stew of sleep and dreams, to the alert and aware world of increased logic and order. Take a moment before opening your eyes to see if you can become aware of what is happening during this transition. Observe the images, words, and feelings that come to mind as you cross over from sleep to waking.

catch phrases

When we say, "The answer just dawned on me," we are acknowledging the way good ideas seem to rise with the sun. But, as with dreams, these early morning insights will fade away if we don't catch them. So keep a stack of index cards or sticky notes at your bedside to jot down any inspiring ideas, poetic lines, or surprising solutions you wake with.

first things first

Because of the brain's unique chemistry as we move from sleep to waking, many people find that morning is the ideal time for sketching out possible approaches for a story, a meeting, or a class they'll be teaching. It's also a great time to do crossword puzzles and brain training games. Take advantage of your fresh perspective in the morning by doing tasks that require flexible thinking or creativity first.

• • • • • • • •

MORNING BREATH

A lovely way to wake the body and mind is with some deep, cleansing morning breaths. To begin this 10-breath mini-mediation, which you can do in bed or soon after rising, lie on your back with arms and legs relaxed at your sides, or sit up in such a way that your spine feels long and relaxed. Prepare by shifting your focus to your breath, observing the sensation of air filling your chest, diaphragm, belly, and the front, sides, and back of your body. Now you are ready to begin:

1. With the next three breaths, scan your body from the crown of your head to the tips of your toes. On the inhalation, notice (no judging) what you feel. Which parts of your body feel easeful and which are cranky or creaky? Soften and release on the exhalation.

2. With the next three breaths, notice your thoughts. Don't settle on any particular thought, just notice what you are experiencing right now. Notice on the inhalation, and let go of anything that's not serving you on the exhalation.

3. With the next three breaths, connect with your heart center. Observe the feelings in and around your heart, including any physical sensations, such as breath flowing easily or feeling stuck, as well as thoughts, images, and emotions that are filling your heart. Notice what's residing in your heart on the inhalation, and release any self-judgment or self-criticism (anything that is not self-love) on the exhalation.

4. On your final breath, ask yourself what is your heart's deepest desire? If an answer arises, that's wonderful. If not, that's wonderful, too. Your heart will brighten a bit just from being asked.

Waking up this morning,
I smile knowing there are
24 brand new hours before
me. I vow to live fully in each
moment and to look at beings
with eyes of compassion.

THICH NHAT HANH

ON THE RIGHT SIDE OF THE BED

E ach morning you have an opportunity to hit the reset button — another chance to open your eyes anew to the wonders of being alive. But, instead, some days you wake up "on the wrong side of the bed." You're uncharacteristically grumpy. You feel as though you've been tossed unceremoniously onto the shores of morning, tangled in seaweed and choking on saltwater like someone who barely survived a shipwreck.

The idea that we can wake up on the wrong side of the bed for seemingly no good reason is centuries old and is rooted in the superstitious belief that getting up on the left side, or even stepping out of bed with the left foot, was unlucky.

The truth is that sides of the bed are beside the point. The greatest predictor of waking in good spirits has to do with one thing: Getting enough sleep. But sometimes, despite our best efforts, that's not possible. We don't always have control over how many hours of shut-eye we log, but we can apply positive intention to the process of awakening in the morning — which can do wonders for starting the day on the right foot . . . even if it's the wrong one!

• • • • • • • •

WAKE-UP CALL

Each morning we are blessed with another chance at a fresh start. But it doesn't always feel that way. Here are a few suggestions for making your first moments in the morning just a bit more conscious — and kind.

don't be alarmed

There's no need these days to wake to a jarring, jangling alarm clock. Instead, choose a clock or app you can program to wake you to gentle sounds from nature, a soft crescendo of music, or even brightening light that mimics the sunrise.

label it with love

If your smartphone is also your alarm clock, edit the standard "Alarm" label and use instead a word or phrase that will affirm your intentions: "Feel the Good," "Love," or "Breathe," for example. Let your alarm wake you to wonder!

• • • • • • • •

YAWN AND STRETCH

There's a fancy name for that instinctive act of flexing the spine, stretching the arms overhead, and letting out a good yawn. It's called *pandiculation*, and doing it mindfully is a great way to add some pleasure, plus health benefit, to your wake-up routine. Yawning isn't only for when we're tired or bored. In fact yawning can help you become more alert, too. When you open your mouth wide to yawn, you also stretch your jaw and neck, and stimulate blood flow to the face and head. That nice big inhale and expansive exhale provides oxygen to the brain and cleanses the body of carbon dioxide, letting your mind and body know you're ready for action.

Here are some more ways to wake up feeling exceptionally well.

the pleasure of pandiculation

The key to primo pandiculation is to let the breath guide the body's movements. Locate a small, rising breath at your center and bring your witnessing attention to it as it gradually gains momentum. Feel your spine elongate and flex in response, and allow your limbs to naturally follow suit as the wave of breath fills your entire belly, chest, and torso, then extends to your shoulders, hips, arms, and legs. Enjoy!

GOOD REASONS FOR GETTING UP

There's so much to love about waking up: The residue of wacky, funny, creative, silly dreams circling the outposts of memory. Birdsong. Morning light stretching out across the landscape outside your window.

Make a list of the best things about waking up. Or choose one to describe in depth, being sure to include sensory details, such as smells, textures, sights, flavors, and sounds.

locate joy

Don't wait to feel good — actively search out pleasant feelings when you awaken. Sure, your limbs might be stiff and your joints achy, but if you pause for a moment or two, you'll find points of pleasure (the subtle weight of blankets against your body, the softness of the pillow beneath your head, a relaxed area in your belly). Shine your attention on the good feeling, no matter how small, and allow it to grow as you breathe into it. Go ahead: feel good!

let there be light

Open the blinds and curtains when you wake up. Bright light triggers the brain to release neurochemicals, including serotonin and dopamine, which help you feel fresh and happy.

splash!

Try replacing that first cup of coffee with a bracing morning routine: wash your face with cold water or take a cool shower to bring you to full alertness — but without the sometimes negative effects of caffeine.

salute the sun

Even five minutes of exercise in the morning is enough to signal to your mind that it's time to wake up and start the day. Doing a couple of rounds of sun salutations is one good option. Another way to welcome the sun is to take a brisk morning walk. Being outdoors in the early daylight helps regulate sleep patterns and activates serotonin and other neurochemicals that help you feel good.

diy morning massage

Pamper yourself with a massage in the morning to wake your muscles, get your blood flowing, and get your day off to a delightful start. You don't even need a personal massage therapist. This is a massage you can give to yourself.

Begin by sitting up on a rug or yoga mat. Then, using relaxed pressure, gently knead your skin, starting at the extremities and working your way in toward your center, as follows:

1. Start at the crown of the head and work your way down, massaging the back and sides of the head, face, and neck.

2. Massage one hand at a time, squeezing each finger than working up the hand, wrist, arm, and shoulder.

3. Give yourself a hug, reaching around to massage as much of the upper back as you can comfortably reach. Then work your way forward and massage the front of the chest.

4. Massage one foot at a time, starting with the toes, then the ball and arch, ankle, lower leg, upper legs, and all the way to the hip.

5. Massage your belly with slow, circular strokes, and reach around to massage your lower back and torso.

6. Now lie on your back, hug your knees to your chest, and roll gently from side to side, massaging your spine, back, and the back of your head.

7. Come to stillness, and lie on your back with arms and legs stretched out on the ground in relaxation pose for the length of 3 to 10 slow, easy breaths, as you bask in the glow of self-love and appreciation.

8. When you are ready, roll to your side, and get up slowly.

bright breakfast

We've all heard that breakfast is the most important meal of the day, but what you eat and drink, and how much, is important, too. Consider these tips to eat well and start the day bright and refreshed.

DRINK UP. Drinking two glasses of water before breakfast will help facilitate a gentle cleanse for your body. Sip mindfully, taking a moment to feel grateful for the gift of fresh, clean water, and nourish your spirit along with your body.

THE TIGER IN YOUR TANK. Eating a breakfast featuring healthy fats and proteins (such as eggs, plain or low-sugar yogurt, and all-natural nut butter) will help you cut through morning brain fog. On the other hand, too many carbohydrate-rich foods like cereal, toast, and pancakes will slow you down and make you feel sluggish.

THE SMALL PLATE CLUB. Eating too much in the morning will bog you down, so choose a small plate or bowl at breakfast to help you manage your portions.

• • • • • • • •

WAKEY WAKEY

We wake up countless times each day. We wake up in the morning, of course, but we also wake ourselves from one form of consciousness to another when, for example, we conclude a meditation session or when we shift from day-dreaming to focusing on our work again. We wake up to new understandings and new ideas, too. Each awakening heralds a new beginning and is therefore a moment to celebrate.

wake again . . .

Each time you need a new start today, wake yourself up: When you need a new perspective, or you want to wake from fear into love or from resistance into acceptance, pause, close your eyes, and take a conscious breath . . . or two . . . or three. When you are ready to open your eyes again, smile and feel gratitude for the opportunity to wake up to another new beginning.

. . . and again

Another way to wake up is to seek out beauty or make note of three things that are worth wondering at: a smile, the wagging of a dog's tale, the rich hues of a maple leaf changing colors from green to gold to red, the scent of fresh laundry, a slice of lemon . . .

notice and take note

When do you feel most awake and aware during the day? Take note of the activities, relationships, and thought patterns that make you feel bright as the sun.

*Dreams are
today's answers
to tomorrow's
questions.*

EDGAR CAYCE

epilogue
SOUND SLEEP FOR ALL

As I lie in bed with sleep creeping at the corners of my consciousness, just out of reach, I sometimes find myself feeling heartbroken and angry over the latest news story: a humanitarian crisis, a devastating storm, political unrest, or the most recent mass shooting in a theater, school, or mall. I know I'm not alone in feeling the unsettled nature of the world or even in lying awake sickened and saddened by the suffering and loss that seems brutal and senseless.

In moments like these, I think of others who are also lying awake in the dark, and who, like me, are concerned about the state of affairs in general, as well as for those who are directly affected by the events behind the headlines. I think of the children who've witnessed violence or viciousness that they can't rub from their eyes, and their parents holding wakeful vigils by their bedsides. Then there are all those who can't stop hearing the gunshots, or the explosions, or the screams, or the sirens — even when there is (finally) silence, however brittle it may be. There are still others who won't sleep because the violence lives with them under their own roof or because they can't shake the nightmare of an earlier trauma.

Even on an ordinary day, when only the scandals of minor political players grab headlines, sleep doesn't come easily to us all — nor does it come *equally* to us all. Whether because of homelessness, poverty, domestic violence, street violence, childhood abuse, illness, terrorist threats, or all-out war, far too many people are deprived of a safe environment (in both the physical and psychological sense) in which to rest and sleep.

Not knowing what else to do in the face of this unrest, both political and personal, we "send our love" via social-media posts to those affected, and our leaders and public figures send their well-meaning prayers to the families of those who were slain or are suffering. But we all know prayers and wishes alone are not enough. We want *real* peace and *real* change so everyone can feel safe and protected, enjoy a good night's sleep, and wake to a world that supports safety, comfort, and ease for all.

Then again, when done with sincerity, saying prayers or offering loving thoughts is not a bad place to start. Sending out good thoughts in the form of prayer, wish, desire, intention, imagination, or dream *does* count. Focusing on how we feel and what we want for our world helps keep our hearts open and connected, which is a first and essential step toward creating conditions where seeds of caring, love, and support might someday grow.

• • • • • • • •

SENDING LOVE

One of my favorite ways to soften my own heart and strengthen my ability to empathetically connect with others is *metta*, or loving-kindness, meditation. In this practice, which comes from the Buddhist tradition, we send blessings for happiness, love, safety, and peace for oneself, one's loved ones, friends, and the wider community — eventually including all beings. You can do this meditation during the day sitting up or lying in bed at night. There are many forms of metta meditation, but I've tailored these instructions for lying in bed as you prepare for sleep.

1. Snuggle under the covers, and lie on your back with your hands resting palms down on your abdomen or your heart. Bring your attention to your breath, and affirm that you dedicate your sleep and dreams tonight to the safety and well-being of all people, everywhere.

2. Think about something you love about yourself, and feel your heart fill with appreciation.

3. Direct three to five simple heartfelt wishes to yourself, such as, "May I be happy, may I be loved, and may I live in safety and peace." Repeat these wishes several times, coordinating the phrases with your breath.

4. Now think of someone you love unconditionally, such as a family member or child, and do the same for him or her.

5. Repeat this process of filling your heart with love and extending these wishes to a friend you care about, then an acquaintance toward whom you feel neutral, then to someone with whom you have a difficult relationship or whom you actively dislike, and finally to all people and all beings everywhere.

There's no one set script for this meditation. You can adapt it to make the words meaningful to you. And don't be discouraged if it feels difficult sometimes. Extending loving kindness to all people without exception isn't easy. Be gentle with yourself, and if you get stuck, simply return to directing loving kindness to yourself or someone you love unconditionally. Over time it will become easier. And in the process you'll build your heart's capacity for empathy, love, and, ultimately, for right action.

SLEEPING (AND DREAMING) TOGETHER

Dreams know no boundaries. They speak to everyone, no matter what our language, race, creed, age, or income. They therefore offer us a powerful — and beautiful — way to connect both with our deepest selves and with one another. Consider these ideas for helping you to use dreams to connect in meaningful ways with the wider world.

let it begin with me

One night a month, or more frequently if you like, dedicate your sleep and dreams to creating peace in some area of your wider community, such as your family, your neighborhood, your workplace, or the world. Take a little extra time in the evening to relax and wind down, feeling still and peaceful inside. Think about your dream dedication, and write it in your journal before bed. Pay attention to your dreams to see if they offer guidance or wisdom about the topic you intended to dream about.

the big picture

We are used to looking to our dreams for personal messages, but dreams address larger issues as well. Archetypes are universal symbols in dreams that connect us to collective myths and wisdom. Their appearance reminds us that dreams go beyond our personal concerns and extend to collective issues as well. When you have a dream that seems to be pointing you beyond your individual life to concerns of the wider world, honor that dream in some way, such as by volunteering for something, making a donation to a charity, or doing a random act of kindness for a stranger.

give me shelter

Consider making a donation to a charity, casting a vote, or doing volunteer work for a candidate or cause that supports ending homelessness and giving shelter to those in need of a safe place to sleep. Other causes that help create safety in sleep, and which you might wish to support in some way, are those that advocate for ending domestic violence and putting an end to war and violence of all types.

May you enjoy good nights, good dreams, and countless opportunities to wake well.

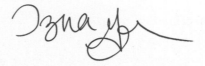

*And so even though we face
the difficulties of today and tomorrow,
I still have a dream.*

MARTIN LUTHER KING JR.

YOUR DREAM TRACKER

Use this dream tracker as an adjunct to your journal to uncover patterns and themes in your dreams. As time goes on, it will provide a quick snapshot or overview of your dream life and can help you reference your complete dream report in your journal as needed.

Copy one of these pages and place it inside your journal, or create a similar chart of your own.

You can use the Notes section to track any additional elements that interest you, such as extraordinary dreams (lucid, precognitive, or big dreams, for instance), the quality of your sleep, medications that might affect your dreams, and other details.

Tracking dreams in this way can also help spark insights into themes that arise both in your dreams and your waking life.

DATE	/	/

DREAM TITLE ....

DREAM CHARACTERS ....

....

....

....

IMAGES/SYMBOLS ....

....

....

PRIMARY EMOTION ....

NOTES ....

....

....

....

....

....

....

DATE   /   /

DREAM TITLE ....

DREAM CHARACTERS ....

....

....

....

IMAGES/SYMBOLS ....

....

....

PRIMARY EMOTION ....

NOTES ....

....

....

....

....

....

....

....

DATE   /   /

DREAM TITLE

DREAM CHARACTERS

IMAGES/SYMBOLS

PRIMARY EMOTION

NOTES

DATE   /   /

DREAM TITLE ....

DREAM CHARACTERS ....

....

....

....

IMAGES/SYMBOLS ....

....

....

PRIMARY EMOTION ....

NOTES ....

....

....

....

....

....

....

....

....

ACKNOWLEDGMENTS
Mutual Dreams

Sleeping may be a private activity, but dreaming up a book requires a concerted collective effort. I would like to acknowledge and express my gratitude for my family of dreamers who are part of the International Association for the Study of Dreams, my students (who teach me so much) at the Institute for Dream Studies, and everyone who has generously shared their dreams with me. I am deeply grateful in particular to these colleagues and friends in the world of sleep and dreams: Betsy Grund, David Kahn, Hermine Mensink, Jane Porter, Justina Lasley, Laura Baughman, Sherry Treadaway Puricelli, Sylvia Green-Guenette, and Ted M. Jones. I also extend my gratitude to my writing community, especially Susan Stinson and the members of the Writing Room at Forbes Library, Rachel Hass, Patricia Lee Lewis, Nerissa Nields, and Naila Moreira.

I would also like to give a joyous shout-out to the powerful friends and dreamers who supported and surrounded me during the writing of this book, including Aja Riggs, Ana Rodriguez, Anita Gallers, Claudia V. Johnsen, Elise Gibson, Grace Welker, Lesléa Newman, Lori Soderlind, Molly Hale, Rachel Kuhn, Riva Danzig, Ruth Anne Lundeberg, and Virginia Pasternak. I am so grateful for my loving family, including Richard and Diane Gover, James Gover, Miranda Sanders, my sister, my niece, and my mother, the late C. Jane Covell, who was a beautiful dreamer. And, for sharing and supporting my dreams, a sweet and special thank you to Louis Moore.

I am so lucky to have the opportunity to work with the dream team of creative, curious, and committed people at Storey Publishing. Special thanks to Hannah Fries and Deborah Balmuth for helping to bring this book into the light of day.

And last but in no way least, I thank the dreams that visit me to encourage, bless, challenge, entertain, instruct, correct, inspire, and delight me.

Index

comfort. *See also* pillow(s)
  bedroom and, 12
  beds and, 10–11
  safe space, 4
connectedness, 73
consciousness. *See also* lucid dreaming
  brain activity states and, 27
  dreaming and, 68
  dreams popping into, 80
  honoring dreams and, 139
  living lucidly and, 134
  mysteries of, 10
  shifting nature of, 28, 101
  waking from forms of, 151
cortisol, 29
counting, 41, 43
creativity. *See also* imagination
  darkness and, 51
  dreams and, 58
  dreamwork and, 63
  pillow art, 35
  waking up and, 142
curtains, 51, 117, 148
cycles, sleep, 27–28

Darkness, 47, 49–51
  bedroom blackout, 51
  sunset and, 26
death, dreams and, 120, 125
decoding dreams, 91–93
  exercise for, 92–93
depression, herbs and, 36
dopamine, 148
Dorveille, 141
dream(s). *See also* nightmares; transcendent dreams
  about, 61–62
  "aha!" moment and, 90
  beliefs about, 72–73
  big, memorable, 125
  children's, 88
  connectedness and, 73

creativity/innovation and, 58
dedication of, 156
dream groups, 88
extraordinary, 124–25
fragments of, 80
gratitude and, 22
honoring your, 139
illogical, 69
'jacking, 90
myths about, 58
precognitive, 125
questions about your, 72, 83
recording, 31
science and, 67–73
themes, 80, 120
waking, 77
word origin, 62
dreaming
  as natural, 57
  prevalence of, 57
  reasons for, 70
dream journal. *See also* journaling
  dream report, 102–5
  keeping a, 80
  words, magic of, 101–2
  Zen and art of, 99–105
dream language. *See* dreamwork
Dream Language (Hoss), 92
dream recall, 75–83
  dream themes and, 80
  factors interfering with, 76
  harvesting dreams, 79–80
  interpretation and, 81–83
  journaling and, 58
  tips for, 76–77
dream report, 102–5
  beyond the basics, 104–5
  headlines for dreams, 102
dream sharing
  conversations and, 87–88
  safety in sharing, 90–91
dream tracker, 159–167

posture, *continued*
  sleeping and, 110, 112
power
  living lucidly and, 137–39
  superpowers, 115, 119
  wisdom and, 137–39
pranayama, 39
prayers. *See* spirit/spirituality
precognitive dreams, 125
prophetic dreams, 36
psychic dreams, 36
psychotherapy, nightmares and, 116

Quiet. *See also* silence
  meditation, 53
  quiet time, 52

Rapid eye movement (REM) sleep. *See* REM sleep
reading
  bedside, 2–3
  scary stories, 119
  soothing stories, 13
reflection
  dream report and, 102, 104–5
  dream sharing and, 91
  gratitude and, 63
  morning, 85
  reacting versus, 86, 134, 137
  writing prompts and, 132
relaxation
  aromas and, 13
  DIY morning massage and, 149
  dream scents and, 36
  energy centers and, 25–26
  techniques, 43
relaxation pose (*savasana*), 43, 108, 112
REM sleep, 68, 69, 71, 128
rest, productive, 44–45
routines
  alert/alarm for, 30
  alertness and, 148

changing, 3
getting settled and, 38
nighttime, 21

Safety
  safe space, 4, 117–18
  sharing dreams and, 90–91
sanctuary for sleeping, 12–13
savasana, 43, 108, 112
scary dreams. *See* nightmares
scents. *See* aromas
schedule, 21. *See also* routines
science, dreams and, 67–73
seratonin, 43, 148
shades and blinds, 51, 117, 148
shared dreams, 125
silence(s), 47
  peace in, 52–54
  sleeping environment and, 54
  between words, 52
skeletal dream exercise, 96–97
sleep/sleeping
  dreaming brain and, 68
  geometry of, 27–28
  REM sleep, 68, 69, 71, 128
  survival and, 19
sleep cycles, 27–28
sleep hygiene, 11, 24
sleepiness
  falling asleep and, 41
  getting sleepy, 19–22
sleep masks, 51
sleepwear, 2, 25, 51
snoring, 54
social media, 31, 42
songs, soothing, 15–17
spirit/spirituality. *See also* meditation
  enlightenment and, 7, 65, 107–8
  feeding your spirit, 21–22
  prayers and, 22, 34, 118, 154
  "third eye" and, 112
stillness, 47, 48–49

More Inspiration for Mindful Living
from Tzivia Gover

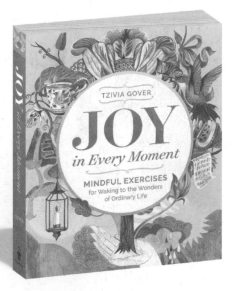

Short inspirational essays and dozens of simple, creative exercises guide you in bringing mindfulness and gratitude into every aspect of your daily routine, including time spent at home, at work, with family, and alone.

"Our lives are the sum total of the moments we spend and savor. Tzivia Gover offers multiple ways to make the most of each moment and, consequently, of our lives."

— Tal Ben-Shahar, author of *Being Happy*

"Immensely practical and written for regular people, this book can fit into even the busiest life."

— Sharon Salzberg, author of *Real Happiness*

"Gover counsels better living through a thoughtful embrace of the ordinary."

— *The Columbus Dispatch*

"[Gover] aims to help readers discover joy at home, work, alone, or in celebration with others with suggestions that range from counting blessings and gardening to journaling and unplugging devices."

— *Library Journal*

"A basic primer on positive thinking — using small, creative ways to get away from negativity and find happiness in the routines of daily life."

— *Daily Hampshire Gazette*